Brooklyn Beginnings

A Geriatrician's Odyssey

May 2010

With Best Wishes
to Melanie,

[signature]

Brooklyn
Beginnings

A Geriatrician's Odyssey

Michael Gordon, MD

iUniverse, Inc.
New York   Bloomington

iUniverse books may be ordered through booksellers or by contacting:

iUniverse
1663 Liberty Drive
Bloomington, IN 47403
www.iuniverse.com
1-800-Authors (1-800-288-4677)

ISBN: 978-1-4401-3423-4 (sc)
ISBN: 978-1-4401-3425-8 (dj)
ISBN: 978-1-4401-3424-1 (ebook)

Library of Congress Control Number: 2009929604

Printed in the United States of America

iUniverse rev. date: 05/20/2009

To my parents and grandparents:
You provided me with the desire to learn, teach, and explore
the world.
And to my children, Neta, Amir, Talia, and Eytan:
All of my learning, teaching, and exploration
have inspired me to be the best parent that I can be.

"How wonderful, how very wonderful the operations of time, and the changes of the human mind!" And following the latter train of thought, she soon afterwards added: "If any one faculty of our nature may be called more wonderful than the rest, I do think it is memory. There seems something more speakingly incomprehensible in the powers, the failures, the inequalities of memory, than in any other of our intelligences. The memory is sometimes so retentive, so serviceable, so obedient; at others, so bewildered and so weak; and at others again, so tyrannic, so beyond control! We are, to be sure, a miracle every way; but our powers of recollecting and of forgetting do seem peculiarly past finding out."

—Fanny Price in *Mansfield Park*,
by Jane Austen, 1814

Foreword

Looking back on one's life and attempting to find meaning in it is something that most people do, but what constitutes significance is a very personal matter and varies from person to person, and perhaps even from time to time in an individual's lifetime. I undertook the task of trying to capture and communicate some of the important experiences in my life in order to help me understand myself as a child, father, husband, brother, and physician, and understand how I became who I am, personally and professionally. The interplay of all these roles has given me the opportunity to grow and develop the attributes that I see as meaningful both in my life and to those who are closest to me.

I have always been interested in stories. As a youngster, I loved to read, and I loved to listen to the stories told by my maternal grandmother with whom I shared a bedroom along with my younger sister, Diti, during my early childhood years in Brighton Beach in Brooklyn. Grandmother's tales of experiencing pogroms in Lithuania, and then coming to America as a teenager to work in the garment industry, set the stage for what became my life-long curiosity and a love of a good story, be it book or movie. My love of writing developed over time during my school days, but became more pronounced during my first travels in Europe and then during my medical studies when I would use letters to my parents and to my closest friend, Chuck Stickney, to record my adventures. When I look at these letters now, most of which were preserved for me, I recognize my love for the narrative. During my professional career, I always looked at each patient within the context of "the story" of that person, often taking extra time out of my typical clinical role to come to know my patients beyond their clinical concerns. Extensive travel gave me life experiences that are part of an extended narrative with subtexts and nuances that seem to entertain, whether I write the story or tell it.

The opportunity to write the narratives of pieces of my life on a professional basis came out of the encouragement of my colleague and friend, Dr. Mark Clarfield, who, after hearing about my experiences of the Six-Day War that took place while I was visiting my sister who was a Peace Corps worker in Tunisia, encouraged me to write them down. From this support came my first narrative published in *The Medical Post*, Canada's leading newspaper for physicians. From then on, a series of editors with whom I worked encouraged me to submit articles that often reflected my past experiences and observations. The readership seemed eager and pleased to read these, and colleagues and friends would comment on how engaging, insightful, and entertaining they were. The writing for me was always exhilarating as the experience became once again vividly reproduced in my mind and then captured into words.

It was the culmination of these writings, plus the encouragement of friends and my eldest daughter Neta, that led me to write this book. Neta helped me with an article that became part of the first chapter of *Brooklyn Beginnings*. My search for a title that reflected the essence of the book and the nature of its content was the result of a short, sofa-based discussion with my wife Gilda Berger, who came up with the title as one that captured who I am and what this book is about. My long-time friend and medical school flat-mate Steve Imber provided one of the cover photographs.

I was initially quite reticent about undertaking such a project, and, after writing some introductory chapters, showed them to Trish Staples, a colleague from work who had edited some professional articles of mine. I trusted her to tell me honestly whether I should keep writing. Her unbridled enthusiasm, which was then echoed by my friends Chuck Stickney and Mark Clarfield, convinced me to complete the manuscript. I wanted to do so, if for no other reason, that my children, Neta, Amir, Talia, and Eytan, would have something to refer to should they want to know some of the details of my life when I may not be in a position to tell them personally.

Finally, I'd like to offer my gratitude to Susan Hendricks, who undertook to edit the manuscript and transform it into its final version, which I believe truly captures what I wanted to say to my readers. We never met in person; however, our e-mail communications gradually helped us know each other beyond the professional editor-author relationship, which, I believe, enhanced the final version of the manuscript and resulted in my deep appreciation of her talents and insights.

These reflections are selective and are not quite an autobiographical telling of the stories, but, rather, a mixture of memoir and probably less-than-perfect recollections of seminal, emotion-laden, amusing, profound, and poignant experiences of my life. I have changed the names of some of the characters where I felt that issues of privacy and confidentiality must be respected.

I feel honored and grateful that I have been able to study and then practice medicine in the wonderfully challenging and supportive environments that provided the experiences captured in the stories told in the book.

I hope that all who read *Brooklyn Beginnings*—including

the general readership as well as family and friends who know me personally, and colleagues, patients, and their families who have known me in my professional role—find the book both entertaining and insightful, and that it will help expand their understanding, not just of my world and experiences, but of their own as well.

Table of Contents

Chapter 1

What's in a Name?

During a medical evacuation, the wounded are loaded into the helicopter as the pilot makes circular hand signs to hurry so that we can take off, always in a lateral and upward, gut-wrenching fashion to avoid ground fire. Soon, we are circling the hospital's seaside helicopter landing pad. It is 1973, and this will be my last reserve duty as an Israeli Air Force doctor before leaving for Canada. The din of the rotors fills the air as I make sure the two soldiers are secure and all IV lines are taped in place. I check the identification tags of the wounded again against my medical report and sign the medical evacuation forms as we are close to landing. I write my name at the bottom—Michael Gordon, MD—in grade-one-level Hebrew and then below it in English so that I can be identified if further information is needed later on.

I know the drill. I have done helicopter evacuations before. As we touch the landing pad, the wounded soldiers are expertly extracted, moved to gurneys, and rushed to the emergency receiving area. We take off back toward the Lebanese border from where we had come. As we lift off, my identification tag falls to the outside of my flight suit and there, on both halves of the double metal tag, is my name in Hebrew above my military identification number. I push the tag inside my suit as I look out the side windows of the helicopter. I scan this new Rambam Hospital in Haifa, next to the older beachside building where I spent a month as a medical student in obstetrics and gynecology in 1965, and later spent time as an intern in 1967. That first summer month at Rambam, which led inextricably to the current moment in a military evacuation helicopter in Israel, was the result of my name and its history.

It all started with my family name—Gordon—clearly of Scottish origin. As a child, I puzzled over where my name came from as I knew all my grandparents were from somewhere in Eastern Europe. I shared a bedroom with my maternal grandmother during my childhood years and knew she came from a small village in Lithuania. She told me about the murderous pogroms, about her coming to New York as a teenager to enter the garment business, and about becoming a lady garment workers' union organizer. But, of course, her name was not Gordon; that was my father's family name. His father had come from the same small village as my grandmother. When I was about nine years old, I asked him what our name had been before it was changed to Gordon. Most of my friends knew that their names had been changed when their parents or grandparents came from Europe (from rather long names ending in *ovich* or *owitz* or *osky*).

"Gordon has always been our name. My great-grandfather was a Gordon, even in the old country."

I pondered this, and some years later verified the story with my father's oldest brother's wife, while we were both attending a bar mitzvah; she had married into the Gordon family in Lithuania before they immigrated to America. Because of the name, I was a curiosity among my friends.

I had decided on a pre-med curriculum and, following the mesmerizing lectures of a world-traveling professor during my third year of university, decided to take a six-month leave from university and travel in Europe. Our neighbors attempted to convince my parents that undertaking such an apparently frivolous and potentially dangerous idea was crazy; nevertheless, my parents supported the trip. My father, who had worked during the day and studied at night school during the depression and experienced the very restrictive war years working as a department of defense civilian engineer, confided in me, "I always wanted to travel around Europe."

On my return from a six-month meander around Europe, I decided to try and study medicine overseas. I raised the subject to my parents, and, in keeping with their openness of spirit, they encouraged me. After all, some years before they had undertaken a six-week, cross-America trip with me, my sister, and our dog Bingo. We camped all over the country— sleeping in the station wagon, on the ground under the stars, or in a small tent—experiencing a world that most people in our situation could only dream about.

The neighbors were aghast, for they knew that I was a good enough student to get into an American medical school. Why would I want to study overseas? How could my parents allow such a plan? I applied to every reputable medical school in Europe and the United Kingdom. The son of our family dentist's neighbor was attending the medical school at the University of St. Andrews in Scotland, so I made sure I applied to that institution as well. The responses were all positive, but indicated that a place would likely not be available until the fall of 1962, a year and a half away. This meant I would finish my fourth year at Brooklyn College and then enter their first year, unfortunately losing some of the benefits of my pre-med training and adding two years to my studies.

The summer after I returned from my European trip was quiet. I helped my father with his early morning newspaper route, which provided supplementary income to our family. I also took a couple of afternoon summer school philosophy and literature courses at Brooklyn College to make up for some of the credits I was missing because of my term abroad traveling around Europe.

Our home was very close to Brighton Beach, and I had ample opportunity to swim on weekday mornings. The languid, hot, and sticky days spent on the beach with my mother during my childhood, and later on with school friends and neighbors, were integral to the development of my childhood identity. People came from all over New York to spend a day at the beach that, for most of my childhood years, I could see from my apartment window and, now, could easily walk to in less than ten minutes. While it was not too crowded on weekdays, by the weekend it would swell with people using their blankets or chairs to keep them off the hot, white, very fine sand, and sometimes umbrellas to diminish the burning effect of the blistering sun.

The beach scene left a lasting impression on my growing up. The smell of food permeated the air. It seemed everyone was either feeding children or eating picnic lunches, ice cream, cold drinks, soft pretzels, and hot knishes (a baked or fried Jewish snack food consisting of a filling, such as potato, that is covered with dough). These were sold by beach vendors who, while bellowing out what delicacies they were selling, carried their goods in Styrofoam containers. They used dry ice to keep their ice cream cold; clouds of white "smoke" billowed out every time they opened their coolers, delighting the children. Lucky children would sometimes be given a piece of the dry ice, and they would immerse it in water and gleefully watch the small white piece bubble away, furiously producing billows of white smoke.

One late August day when I arrived home from a swim, there was a telegram waiting for me. It was unexpected and exciting. Telegrams were unusual and always worrisome in those days. In the era before e-mail and cell phones, telegrams were often purveyors of either bad news such as the serious illness or death in a loved one, or good news such as congratulatory wishes at weddings. Receiving a telegram was not an ordinary event. I was still dripping wet from my swim at the beach and danced from one foot to the other in excitement and dread as I opened the envelope.

A place had become available at the University of St. Andrews in second year, and the registrar deemed that my pre-medical courses would be accepted in lieu of the first year of studies. I was so excited I did not know where to go: the house was empty, and there was no one around I could share the good news with—especially in a wet bathing suit. Ultimately, my parents came home and, after digesting the news, they agreed to my going, knowing that it would mean my being very far away and that we would not see each other very often as transatlantic travel was quite expensive, and we did not have a lot of money.

In the fall of 1961 I settled in Dundee, an impoverished remnant of the industrial revolution. Many of the tenement houses were covered in a layer of soot from the coal burning that served as their major source of heat. That, along with the gray skies and many days of rain, drizzle, and mist, gave the town of 180,000 people a habitually bleak appearance until the sun came out. Then, everything seemed glorious as the greenery glistened, the light played on the cobblestone streets, and the townsfolk's faces broke into smiles as they said, in their particular Dundee Scottish accent, "Lovely day, isn't it?"

Being an outgoing person, I made friends with classmates and students from other faculties at the university. Most of my friends had never really known an American other than the occasional tourist or those they met during their own overseas travels. Our cultural differences soon became evident: they did not understand the eagerness with which I undertook my studies. During the first few days of anatomy lectures, I raised my hand to ask a question. The professor looked at me with apparent astonishment, stopped his talk, and asked me what I wanted. After he answered and continued lecturing, I raised my hand again and heard a shuffling of feet from my classmates. Following the lecture, Doug and Ian, two of the local Dundee fellows, explained to me, "The whole trick is to get through without any of the profs knowing who you are—no one raises a hand in class!" Soon after, having just bought *Gray's Anatomy*, which was tucked heavily under my arm, I met Doug and Ian on the High Street. They looked at the book and said in their broad Dundonian Scottish accent, "What's that?" "*Gray's Anatomy*," I answered, "the book the prof mentioned." They burst into laughter, "Goodness! Are you daft? The exam is not for one and half years!" said Doug. "Why buy it now?" said Ian. They could not have known my propensity for always being well prepared in my studies or way ahead in deadlines, a trait I have had throughout all my years of study and work.

Between Christmas, Easter, and summer breaks, I had almost five months of vacation per year. I took advantage of my proximity to Europe and planned my travels, the very reason for studying overseas. Cheap travel was available to me as a member of the International Medical Students' Association, and I could match it to places almost anywhere in the world where I might complete the clinical experience required of the degree. One of the trips I planned in 1965 was to Athens, Greece, for an orthopedic and emergency room experience, and then on to Haifa, Israel, for obstetrics and gynecology. I had not yet developed any great interest in Israel, and I didn't have much knowledge of the history of the country—or any Zionistic inclinations—but I did have an interest in the Holocaust and the history of the Second World War, about which I had read a great deal. My grandmother had visited Israel in the early '50s with her Yiddish choir and came back imbued with the country. Based on all of this, I felt I should go, not just out of curiosity, but to honor her memory.

On the journey south toward Athens that May in 1965 to arrive in time for a one-month rotation in June at a large Athens public hospital, I started reading a book on the history of Russia, which was written by a Scottish historian. In one chapter the name Gordon was mentioned in reference to a Russian Jew. Incredibly, the footnote clarified my heritage and roots. In great detail it described the mercenary Scottish general, Patrick Gordon, who successfully fought for Czar Peter the Great. As compensation for battle victories, he was given land in the area my ancestors had come from, some of whom took his name, partly in recognition of his special relationship to the Czar and because he became the landlord of these *shtetles* (small Jewish villages).

Later that summer in Israel, I would have my first medical contact with Holocaust survivors in the obstetrics and gynecology department where I was working. They were being treated for Holocaust-related diseases, including infertility. Although in New York I had seen a few of my grandmother's Eastern European friends with numbers on their arms, this was my first encounter in a medical role with survivors of Hitler's concentration camps.

Within a few days of visiting Israel and starting work at the hospital, much like I might do at home in Brooklyn, I went to the nearby beach. As I walked on the white sand, a great sea of people speaking Hebrew enfolded me while, directly in front of me, was a mother feeding a banana to her child. A peculiar feeling of familiarity washed over me as I recalled those first few days of meeting the patients, the doctors, the vendors, and the people on buses or those walking in the streets. Past and present drew into one as I thought, *These are my people*. It was a powerful, engulfing sense that I had never experienced anywhere or anytime previously. I traveled the country on weekends during the month that followed, re-experiencing this feeling of kinship over and over again. I knew I had to return some day soon.

The chance to return to Israel came, oddly enough, during my final exams in June 1966. I entered the room for my *viva* (oral) in obstetrics and gynecology, not my best subject. The professor was my examiner. He was a large man and towered over most of us when he directed our examinations in his clinics.

He looked at me and said, "You're the Yank, aren't you? With a name like Gordon, surely you must be Scottish."

The clock keeping the ten-minute oral examination time was moving along. With my eye on it, I answered, "Yes, I am the Yank, but my name, although Scottish, has Jewish Lithuanian roots. If you have a moment, I can explain."

His already rose-colored face brightened, and he replied, "Please do."

I spun out the story of my heritage. Two more minutes passed as I spoke of the Czar, and another two as I emphasized General Gordon's role. Explaining the *shtetle* and the taking of names took me to the beginning of the last minute.

The professor suddenly looked at his watch and said, "Oh dear, oh dear; time has flown. Give me three signs or symptoms of preeclampsia."

I carefully and deliberately counted out the answers—"high blood pressure, swelling of the legs with rapid weight gain, and protein in the urine"—finishing just as the minute hand crossed the ten-minute mark.

He stood up, beaming, and shook my hand. As I left the room, I heard him murmur to himself, "Very good. Very good."

That "very good" resulted in my winning the five-hundred-pound prize in obstetrics and gynecology, much to the surprise of my classmates. Following my completion of a six-month stint as a house officer (intern) in medicine at Aberdeen City Hospital, I obtained permission from the professor to use the money to return to Haifa for an internship in obstetrics and gynecology. ("Medicine" in European medicine is the equivalent of "general medicine" in the United States.) I was now on my way to Israel, happy to revisit Haifa's Rambam Hospital for some months of training.

Toward the end of an extraordinary personal and clinical experience, I visited a kibbutz on the Negev border, which abutted the Gaza Strip in Egypt. There I met Indian troops who were serving with the United Nations. A week later, Egypt's President Nasser unilaterally removed these troops, and I left Israel to visit my sister Diti, who was serving with the Peace Corps in Tunisia. It was in the small town of Hammam Sousse in Tunisia that I experienced the Six-Day War. For the first two and a half days, all I could hear on the battery-powered shortwave radio were Arab-language reports and an English-language broadcast from Egypt. Diti could understand, and she translated the depressing news from the Arabic. The English broadcasts came every few hours and were very clear in their details of the destruction of Israel. The BBC was scrambled, so there was no way of hearing any other information.

Incredibly, I managed to find batteries in a bicycle store, for there were none in all the electrical shops. To the surprise of the owner, I bought his whole supply. The next day's local newspapers were full of stories of Israel's destruction, as explained to Diti by those in her school who read the Arabic to her. The people who had become "my people" might disappear in the fire of war. On a visit to Sousse on the second day, we noticed many armed soldiers. A street vendor told Diti that they were Algerian troops on their way to the war "over there—far away." I ran the dial on the shortwave radio back and forth all night on the day the war broke out and again on the second day and night, which was June 6. That night, as I was slowly moving the dial, I heard very distantly, a song, with guitar accompaniment, which I recognized as Hebrew.

The music stopped and a voice came on the air. My knowledge of the language was rudimentary, but the voice sounded calm. Then I recognized that it was the news being read, although I could not understand the details. I heard the word *maot* followed by the word *migim*, which I surmised was the Russian aircraft used by Egypt and Syria. I knew that, since *mea* was a hundred, *maot* must mean hundreds. This was followed by the word *shtemeser*, which I knew meant twelve, followed by the word, *miragim*, which I knew to be the Mirage, the Israeli fighter jet supplied by France. After the news, music started again, and the reception became distant and replete with static. I went to sleep hoping I had understood enough Hebrew to know that things could not be all that bad. The next morning, the BBC made it through and announced the clearer reporting of the war. Israel had not been destroyed, though the war was raging on at least two fronts—Egypt and Syria—and Israeli tanks seemed to be rushing towards the Suez Canal.

Two days later, I flew to Paris and then to London where Steve, my flatmate from medical school, lived. By this time it was known that Jordan had entered the war but had lost their stranglehold on Jerusalem, and the West Bank had been taken over by the Israelis. The last battle going on was for the Golan Heights, which was in full force by the time I arrived in London that Friday, June 9. The news was sketchy, but Israel clearly had survived so far. Steve and I tried vainly to get to Israel to volunteer. Then, suddenly, on Saturday morning while we were walking through Hampstead Heath where a cricket game was being played, the war ended. I left the next day for the United States, and each of us vowed to meet again in Israel.

Two years later, in the fall of 1969, I arrived in Haifa by ship from Greece with my Israeli wife, Yael, having left America in 1968 for Canada for one year of medical residency training. After a three-month late-honeymoon journey through Europe, I was setting foot in Israel again, this time as a married man. I had met Yael just prior to the Six-Day War, during my five-hundred-pound-prize visit, the result of the story of my Scottish name! Now, four years later in 1973, I was bringing wounded Israeli soldiers to the helicopter pad of the new Rambam Hospital, which now dwarfed its older hospital counterpart, the place where, in 1965, as a medical student, I had delivered my first Israeli baby.

Chapter 2

An Accident of Fate

By the time I was an intern at the Aberdeen City Hospital in 1966, I had given up my original plan to be a general practitioner, as family doctors were called at that time. Like many medical students, as I undertook each module of exposure and training, I was either turned off completely of ever thinking of that field of medicine, or grabbed with fascination and the imaginary contemplation of life as an "...ologist" of one sort or another.

I contemplated many fields as I moved up through pre-clinical to clinical training. My fascination with microbiology and infectious disease was encouraged by fantastic teachers in the field; my love of things technical, like microscopes; the major advances in antibiotics; and Paul de Kruif's book, *Microbe Hunters*. I had read it during the first trip I took as a medical student—a journey to Copenhagen during Christmas break after the fall session of first-year medical school classes that began in 1961. It was because of an experience in Copenhagen during my undergraduate junior year abroad in 1960 that I had decided in the first place to pursue my studies overseas. By chance, during that visit, I had been adopted by a group of female Danish medical students.

Our meeting had been fortuitous that late fall of 1960 and was triggered by circumstances of travel. I had meandered though Europe from early summer in a small Renault Dauphine, the deal being that purchasing a car in Europe and then bringing it back duty-free because it was used was financially advantageous. This roller-skate-sized car was a zippy little thing and, compared to my father's American cars I had driven during my adolescent years, was like a toy, yet it flew along the narrow roads of Europe like a charm. I started off from France in late June, studied French intensively for a month in Lausanne, Switzerland, traveled as far south as Italy, and then headed northward through the mountains of Austria. I had an urge to do something unusual after having studied French, so I toured Italy for a month with a university classmate during the second month of the summer in order to appease the anxieties of my parents who were concerned about me traveling alone in Europe. After a month of camping, staying at hostels in Italy, and seeing many churches and museums, I dropped Eliot off at the train station in Milan so he could start on his journey back to Brooklyn. Once he left, I felt liberated, no longer having to check in with another person and come to an agreement before making plans.

I passed through the lush, green mountains and small villages of Austria. I visited Salzburg and then went on to Vienna, where I discovered that you could go to the state opera house for about twenty cents if you were willing to wait in line in the afternoon for "rush" seats. I stayed in a lovely and hospitable student hostel near the Vienna Woods, where I came across an advertisement for Erwin Leiser's newly released film, *Mein Kampf/Adolph Hitler*. I already had an interest in the history of the Holocaust from reading, so I decided to catch the afternoon show. The theater was almost empty. In front of me sat two fellows in their very late teens. During the scenes depicting the rise and triumphs of Hitler, they cheered with obvious joy. More difficult for me to endure was their behavior during the final concentration camp scenes where Jewish bodies were being buried in mass graves: then, they laughed loudly and jabbed each other with apparent glee.

In the knapsack at my feet was the eight-inch hunting knife that I used when traveling for cutting bread and cheese and for opening cans—a common practice for students staying in youth and student hostels. Livid with rage, I slid my hand inside the knapsack and fingered my knife, wondering if I should brandish it threateningly as the film came to a close. I left the theater behind the pair and followed them for about fifteen minutes through the narrow side streets of Vienna, wanting to stop them, threaten them with my knife, and explain how horrible the Nazi war crimes were. I wanted to ask them how they could laugh at such atrocities. My German was rudimentary and really more a mixture of German and Yiddish. I was struggling in my head as to how to explain my actions, knowing that, without such an explanation, my knife-wielding threats would be meaningless. They moved out of my reach, and I realized I could not adequately explain my actions. Moreover, I would likely be charged with assault. I slipped the knife, which I had been holding upright at the opening to my knapsack, back into its deeper pocket.

As they disappeared around a corner, I decided at that moment that I wanted a Jewish star to hang on the chain that I had found a few weeks earlier on an Italian beach. It was made of rather heavy eighteen-karat Italian gold. I had been wearing it without anything on it, having given the St. Christopher's medal that originally had been attached to it to a little girl walking on the beach near me. I entered the first and rather large jewelry store that I came upon and, in my broken German, which was laden with Yiddish pronunciation, explained that I wanted to buy a *stern* (German for "star"). When I was shown a gold five-pointed star, I said, "No, a *Judisha stern* and drew a *Mogen David* on a sheet of paper. The saleslady blanched and said in understandable English, "We have them no more." I went from jeweler to jeweler and had the same experience in various iterations, which ranged from apparent dismissive ignorance to mildly sympathetic disbelief that I would even ask.

I was growing angry. The images of the film kept coming back to me and, now, as I associated a Jewish star in some symbolic way as an act of defiance and expression of identity, I was determined to find one to wear. I had a desire to declare who I was in a way I had not felt necessary to do thus far in my life. Suddenly, I came upon a very small jewelry store on a narrow street. In the display case, along with a number of gold charms clearly intended for charm bracelets, was a small *Mogen David* surrounded by a circle of gold. I could not believe it. I entered the store and asked to see it. When I asked the price and showed him the chain that I wanted it attached to, the proprietor, a bespectacled man in his late forties, inquired in mixed English and German about its intended recipient. I answered, *Fur mir*, trying to use my best, but broken, German and pointed to myself showing him the chain that was around my neck. He said, "Two dollars," and he strung the gold loop of the star onto my chain. I thought I had heard him wrong as it seemed so inexpensive, but, when I took out my Austrian schillings, he would accept only the equivalent of the original quote of two dollars. He smiled at me as I thanked him profusely, answering his question about my origins, explaining that I was originally from New York but my grandparents were from Lithuania. I left the store veritably coveting the newly purchased star.

As I drove from Austria through Germany, I began to run out of money. Even though the Renault was small and gas efficient, the cost of running it was substantial for my poor budget. The normal method of transferring money in those days was via the American Express offices, which also had a *poste restante* service through which travelers like me could pick up mail. The problem was that, if you changed your itinerary, redirecting mail from one *poste restante* to another was not easy and often very time-consuming. Sometimes you had to follow your original itinerary based simply on the need to be able to stay in touch by mail and receive money transfers.

I arrived in Hamburg, having already spent a few nights sleeping on the backseat of the Renault—a bit of a squeeze even for someone who was just 5' 8"—so I could keep money for gas and food. I had become quite Spartan in my habits. As usual, my creative language skills and my childhood recollections of Yiddish (honed during my travels through Austria to sound more like German) gave me the courage to approach some of the people I saw while walking around Hamburg's central train station. I could usually find the train station no matter where I traveled since, invariably, It is located at the center of European cities. To get directions to the central train station, one of the first German phrases I learned was, *Wo ist de Bahnhof?* By following the *links* and *rechts* in the directions I would receive, I would eventually get to where I was going. Along this route, I picked up other directional communicative jewels, such as *erste* and *zweite* for "first" and "second" and *strasse* for "street," so, if I asked often enough, I was usually able to reach my destination.

After resting a while in the early morning sun on the lawn in front of the huge, architecturally ornate and massive train station, I managed to approach a youngish adult who looked reliable and explain to him that I was a student who was running out of money and needed to find a way to make some rather quickly. He directed me to the flower, fruit, and vegetable market behind the station. I entered this huge hall teeming with vendors and merchants and boxes and crates of flowers and produce. After a few minutes and various turndowns, I was told by a flower vendor to bring in boxes of cut flowers recently arrived from the south and put them in vats containing water. Without even asking about pay, I did this for over an hour, managing in the process to become thoroughly wet. The job completed, the vendor paid me an amount in deutschmarks that would buy me about five liters of gas which, in the Renault, would take me a fair distance. As I walked around looking for another job, a man who looked to be in his late thirties or early forties grabbed me by the arm and asked me in German if I wanted to work, to which I gave a resounding "*Ya!*" He directed me in German (which I now semi-understood) to a pickup truck and told me we were going to load something into his truck. (I could not understand initially what *zwiebel* were, but when we arrived at the destination no more than a fifteen-minute drive away, I realized from the odor coming from the railway cargo car that they were onions!)

The man who took me for work asked me my name, which I knew how to pronounce with a German inflection. He pointed to himself and indicated his name to be Adolf. A momentary shudder ran down my spine; here I was at a cargo train in Germany with cars like those that carried Holocaust era Jews to their deaths at Auschwitz, and I was working with man whose name was Adolf. My recently acquired star was hidden under my shirt, and I made sure it stayed there. He looked at me, then grabbed a woven bag into which he threw onions, placed it on a scale, and, when he had added enough more onions to make five kilograms, pulled at a wire, tied the bag, and threw it into his truck. Speaking slowly and deliberately so I would understand, he indicated to me that I should do the same. The smell of the onions filled the air and my lungs. I started to work, got into the rhythm, and heard from him after about ten minutes, "*Zehr gut!*" with a wink as he picked up another sack. We continued throughout the morning with a break about halfway through. He pulled out some bread and cheese and a thermos of coffee, poured some for me and beckoned me to eat, cutting the loaf and the cheese with a large utility knife that he had in an old metal lunch box.

"*Fon vo comst du?*" he asked, to which I could respond easily—"*Hamerica.*"

"*Ah, zehr gut; ein student?*"

"*Yah, ich vilst studeren Medizin,*" I replied, formulating the answers from the Yiddish and German that were now getting all mixed up in my mind. We finished eating and started loading more onions. We finished at about noon, having found a rhythm in which we both did our parts, with the result that the railway car's load had been quickly bagged into five-kilogram sacks and stacked neatly in his truck.

"*Fertig,*" he said as we closed the railway car with a loud clank that jarred my nerves and caused a flashback to reverberate through my mind of film footage I had seen of Jews being removed roughly from railway cars, the sliding doors slamming shut on their hopes of freedom. The image passed as we jumped into the truck and drove back to the vegetable market which, by now, was full of merchants buying goods for their stores and restaurants. He backed the truck into a dock and we unloaded the sacks. Adolf took out a wad of money, peeled off a considerable number of bills, and gave them to me. Even without actually counting them, I could see that it was a generous and welcome amount. He slapped me on the back and held out his hand, "*Sehr gut—auf Wiedersehen,*" to which I replied, "*vielen dank, vielen dank,*" as I shook his hand firmly in sincere thanks.

I found my Renault where I had parked it not far from the train station, looked at my map, and searched the streets for the one that led to the autobahn north. I would be going to Copenhagen through Germany and then to Jutland in Denmark. Preferring not to immediately spend all the money I had just made, before I entered the highway I filled the tank only halfway with gas, knowing that I would encounter gas stations frequently on the autobahn. I felt a wave of satisfaction; not only had I had managed with my broken German to find work and actually earn some money, more importantly, I had connected to a German man of an age that meant he would have lived through World War II, maybe even have served as a very young soldier in the German army. Adolf had shaken my hand and shared his lunch with me; it had been a strange and somewhat eerie sensation. I wondered to myself what he would have said had I told him I was Jewish. I stayed overnight in a German youth hostel not far from the Danish border, tired from the work but happy to have what seemed to be enough money to get me to Copenhagen.

I continued north toward the Danish-German border, where on its far side, just past the passport check, a young Danish soldier in uniform was thumbing a ride. I loved picking up hitchhikers, and, in those days, it was not considered dangerous. I had picked up many hitchhikers during the trip and used each opportunity to learn about them and their experiences. A uniformed soldier seemed a safe bet. He was from Copenhagen, so I told him I could take him all the way. His English was quite good, and, as we drove, he gave me a running commentary on the geography and important features of the country—the main point seeming to be that Hans Christian Andersen was from Odense, a major town we passed through as we headed eastward toward the main city. We arrived late in the evening, and I let him off at a train station on the way to the center of the city. Unfortunately, I had not estimated the cost of gas to get to Copenhagen very well and, as I entered the downtown area, realized the gas tank was at a quarter full and I only had about twenty dollars left in my pocket. I found a quiet side street just off what appeared to be the central town square and parked the car, curled up in the backseat, and fell asleep.

The next morning I wandered into the town square, where there seemed to be thousands of people on bicycles. I had never seen so many people on two wheels in my life, including some of the most beautiful women I had ever seen, their skirts hoisted up so that they could pedal comfortably. While I was waiting on a corner, mesmerized by the scene, a lovely woman cyclist stopped at the crosswalk to let me pass. She gave me a smile that set me aglow. I reached the American Express *poste restante*, and, to my horror, there was no mail waiting for me. I had expected a letter from my parents containing a money order, but there was nothing there. I checked the signs on the street where the car, which contained all my belongings, was parked and thought it would be safe to leave it there. While it was full of stuff, it did not look particularly inviting to a potential thief. In any event, I did not have an option. I thought of finding the student or youth hostel, but figured another night in the car would not be that terrible an ordeal, particularly since I was really concerned about my severe shortage of money, not to mention the fact that I had not eaten anything substantial since my arrival, and the stash of crackers, bread, and few pieces of cheese I had bought in Germany was about finished.

I wandered around the city, which was unbelievably beautiful, staring like a waif through bakery windows that seemed to have endless supplies of pastries. They looked as inviting as anything I had ever seen. But I wanted to preserve my meager funds, so I settled for some dark bread and cheese, munching on them as I walked. The central shopping street, the *Strøget*, was closed to cars, which gave a festive atmosphere to the place even though it was midweek. I passed a shop where condoms were displayed in the window—I could not believe it ... they were right out in full view of passersby. I stood outside for a few minutes and noted ordinary men of all ages going in and out the doorway. I could see people behind the counter, showing different kinds of condoms. I entered and asked the woman who was available to serve if she spoke English.

"Yes," she replied, with a smile full of exquisite teeth.

"I would like to know what kind of condoms you have here. I am a visitor."

"From where?" she asked, as she took out a tray from behind her which had on it a dozen types of condoms.

"New York."

"Oh, I have been there with my parents … two years ago; such a wonderful city." She started to casually show me all different kinds of condoms, but my embarrassment clearly overcame me when, out of the corner of my eye, I caught a glimpse of a young man being shown how to put the condom on a rubber model of a penis. I thanked her and left with a hasty, "Sorry, but I have to go!" It was unbelievable—showing condoms rather than keeping them tucked away behind the pharmacist's counter! As a virgin from Brooklyn, with only a theoretical knowledge of the whole business of sex, I clearly had a lot to learn!

That evening, quite cold and hungry, I went into the ABC, a large cafeteria not far from the central town square. It was not very crowded. I bought some hot chocolate and a sandwich, thinking I could stay for a long while with those two items, and sat down. A few tables away sat an attractive young woman—uncharacteristically dark-haired—who was reading a large textbook in English. She was marking it with a pencil, and, as she moved the book, I was able to see that it was the green-covered *Ham's Textbook of Histology*, a text I knew from Brooklyn College. Her eye caught mine, and I momentarily looked away but could not help staring at her and pondering the fact that she was reading a book in English. With all the courage I could muster, I took my meager fare and walked over to her table.

"Is that an English histology textbook you are reading?"

"Yes," came the reply in flawless English. "It is for my histology class. I am called 'Puck,'" she said warmly, "you know—from Shakespeare—but my real name is Ellen. I am a medical student."

"Oh, I'm Michael. I hope to be a medical student one day."

She motioned me to sit down, which I did, placing on the table my almost-finished mug of chocolate and my plate with the few remaining morsels of my sandwich.

After an hour of talking and another cup of chocolate that she bought for me because I was a guest in her country, she asked where I was staying.

"I am sleeping in my car until I get some money," I admitted as I explained my difficulty in not finding any money at the *poste restante*.

"Oh, that is terrible; you cannot sleep in a car. It is cold. You will come to my place. I share it with two other medical students, and there is plenty of room."

I could not believe that she was walking with me to my car. I had to move my possessions from the front seat to make room for her. I had put them there so I could sleep in the backseat. The red nylon sleeping bag was still hanging over the backseat. She directed me to her apartment, which was about fifteen minutes from the town square. The apartment was simply furnished in the Danish contemporary style, and very bright. One of her roommates, Dorte, was at home. After a short explanation by Puck, she pointed to a sofa in the sitting room, where they both agreed I could sleep until some other arrangement could be made. The second roommate, Lizbeth, came in while we were eating some soup. She suggested where I might look for a job but advised me that I must first obtain clearance from the department of health. She said she had time in the morning and offered to take me where we had to go. Like Puck, she too had dark hair, Dorte being the only fair-haired, typically Danish-looking girl amongst the three of them.

Without a question, I was given a TB test and told to come back in two days for it to be read. The staff at the clinic filled out a card for me, explaining that I would need it to work, and sent me on my way. Lizbeth suggested that I just walk downtown and inquire for work in the various shops along the way. Speaking English was common in Copenhagen, and a worker who was fluent in the language could be a good asset with the tourists. She came with me and, when there was a bit of a language problem, Lizbeth would pipe in a few words. Everyone was very nice but had no work to offer. In the meanwhile, I sent an express aerogram to my parents telling them about the money issue. Lizbeth told me not to worry; they could help out, if necessary, until I got some money. Just before noon, we entered a shop with sheepskin slippers of all kinds in the window. The woman at the front greeted me, and, when I told her I was looking for work, asked me to stay while she went to the back. Five minutes later she returned, asking me to follow her. Lizbeth came along and said a few words to the woman in Danish as she followed us through a back door. We were in a small workroom where large tables were piled with sheepskins, and parts of the slippers in stacks ready to be sewn.

"Can you cut accurately with a razor knife?" she asked, showing me what back home would have been called an X-Acto knife. I knew it well from my balsa model–building days and my Brooklyn Technical High School training.

"Sure, I will show you if you give me something to cut."

She handed me a piece of sheepskin with the outline of the slipper sole marked in ink and said, "Cut!" indicating the line. Within minutes of completion, she showed me to a table, pointed to a pile of skins with markings, and said, "You can work here." She named an hourly wage that Lizbeth, with a wink, indicated to me was okay.

The woman in the front who hired me also sewed the slippers. Each time I brought her a pile of cut skins, I spoke to her, having decided I would try speaking in German. I assumed that it might be easier for her than English since, when we first did speak, her English seemed more broken than that of most of the other Danes with whom I had spoken. She acknowledged that she spoke German, and I got into the habit of using that language with her. By evening, I figured I had cut at least a hundred pieces and marveled at how she already had sewn them into slippers and given them back to me so I could stamp the size on the sole and put them together as a pair ready to be boxed.

That evening at the apartment, the girls told me that they were having a bit of a party in my honor, as it was just before the weekend and there were no classes the following day. I had already taken my personal belongings from the car, and my newfound friends had provided me with some storage space so that the sitting room would be unencumbered by my things. By eight o'clock, other students had arrived, each bringing some sort of alcohol or food. The music began playing and everyone started to eat and drink and dance. I told my story quite a few times as each new person spoke to me and I was plied with one Coca-Cola and rum after another. I had never been much of a drinker and told the girls so. They laughed and said, "So, you can be drunk for the first time here, amongst friends." It seemed okay, and, since the Coca-Cola was so sweet, I could barely tell there was rum in the drinks.

The room started thinning out as people left; I began to feel the room spinning, but was still able to dance to the loud rock-and-roll music. Puck had her arms around my neck and started nuzzling into me. I felt myself quite unsteady and told her I needed to lie down a bit. She told me to go into her room as it was quieter than the sitting room. I curled up on her bed, feeling both dizzy and nauseated. I realized I could hardly stand, so I just stayed horizontal. I could hear the voices in the next room, which gradually diminished. And then Puck climbed into bed next to me, in her nightgown, and started pulling off my clothes. She was laughing at me.

"How does it feel to be drunk for the first time?"

"Terrible. I feel like throwing up, but there is nothing

there." I was in my undershorts only as she pulled the covers over the two of us. She put her arms around me and started to kiss my neck. My mind was racing.

Is this going to be it? I thought to myself. *I don't even have a condom. This is Denmark. I know that they have "free love," but what do I do if she gets pregnant?*

My head felt like it would burst. The room was spinning, the orange walls wavering before me. I could feel Puck's hand move under my shorts, but, with all my drinking and all my thinking, I couldn't seem to respond. Puck nuzzled me and continued to caress me.

"Do you know Shakespeare, Puck?" I asked.

She laughed, "Of course. Remember, Hamlet was from Denmark."

"You know, then, the speech of the porter in Macbeth?" Having memorized it in school, and having heard Professor Grebanier in my Brooklyn College Shakespeare course acting out the role in class using his best Shakespearean drunken voice, I started to spout it in an appropriately slurred, rather loud voice. "'Lechery, sir, it provokes, and unprovokes; it provokes the desire, but it takes away the performance,'" to which Puck started laughing uncontrollably. I continued the whole speech, over her laughter, as her hands were still very much in my shorts, and I could think of no other response, finishing grandly with, "it 'equivocates him in a sleep, and, giving him the lie, leaves him.'"

"Puck, I do not think I can do anything. Maybe we can just be friends and not do this. I am still a virgin."

Then I continued to babble away until she gave up and we both fell asleep. In the morning, she had coffee and toast ready for me and told me I had to go fast to get to work. She gave me a little kiss and said, "It was fun last night. What happened has never happened to me before. I want you to come to my house. My parents are nice people. My mother is Danish and my father Jordanian—that is why I have the dark hair and dark eyes." She pushed me out of the door, and I ran most of the way to work, not wanting to be late on my second day.

Two nights later, I got a message from Puck that everyone but Lizbeth was busy with studies or meetings, but that Lizbeth was free to spend the evening with me. We went to a bar and each had a beer—for me it was my first taste of Tuborg. In keeping with my limited drinking experience, I did not know one beer from another but found the taste of this one much better than what I associated with the beer back home. All during our conversation she stared at me and laughed a lot. When we got home, she sat on my sofa while I faced her on a chair, and we listened to some quiet, popular music. She told me about her home in Aarhus, how she had found her roommates, and how much fun studying medicine was; that, in Denmark, they started medical school right out of high school without having to go to university, as was the practice at home, so, in fact, the beginning students were on the young side—she being only twenty years old, a year older than I.

Her legs were crossed, and the upper one moved up and down to the musical beat as she kept staring at me. Finally, she leaned over and kissed me and pulled me to her. This time, at least, I was not drunk, just very nervous. She lay down on her back and pulled me to her and started moving below me. Each time I tried for her skirt she pulled my hand away and said, "Just do this," as she began to move rhythmically below me. I followed suit and could feel and hear her breathing change. Suddenly, she started panting and moaning and then she stopped and put her arms around me. "Again," she said after a few moments. This all being new to me, I tried a little more groping at her breasts and then between her legs, but, again, she pushed my hands away. "Just do this." So I did, and this time I got into it too, with both of us still fully dressed. On the verge myself, I whispered in her ear to let her know.

"Go ahead. It is good," as she moaned very loudly indeed … and then, so did I!

After a while, she got up and straightened her skirt and sweater and leaned over and gave me a kiss.

"Do you want something to eat or drink?"

I was stunned. "I need to go to the bathroom," I said to her, a little awkwardly. There, I cleaned up and marveled at what had just happened. What a force! When I came out, she was preparing some coffee and sandwiches for us. We talked more about medical school. Puck came in an hour later.

"So did you have a nice time?"

Lizbeth answered, "Yes. We went to the Drop In and had a beer."

I just looked at her and Puck who said, "Great. I'm heading to bed—early morning in histology lab tomorrow."

Two weeks later, my money arrived with a letter from my parents at American Express. I told the seamstress that I would be leaving, and she arranged for my pay. It was quite a sum. As I was saying good-bye, she said to me, "You are a very nice boy. By the way, what you are speaking is not really very good German, but I understand it. I used to hear it a lot."

She shook my hand and wished me well. As I left the shop and walked across the street to the bakery with the intention of buying all the pastry I could possibly eat, I thought of her words and wondered how it was that she recognized Yiddish-laden German. I did not go back to ask her, but somehow felt a connection to her. I ate so much pastry I was almost sick, but the rich sweetness of the butter-filled, almond-crusted, and fruit-filled baked goods was heavenly.

The letter that arrived a few weeks later from my father said, "Your mother is very worried about you. She wants you to come home soon. Mrs. Greenspoon keeps telling her that the Danish *shiksas* (non-Jewish women) will get you married and you will never come home." Mrs. Greenspoon was our neighbor who treated her sons as if they were mentally defective, always telling them what to do. She was also the one who told my parents that letting me go to Europe was crazy. Fortunately for me, they had not listened. But now my father's words could not be ignored. *Shiksas*—my fantasy, my dream. Over the remaining weeks, I found a room of my own in which to stay but kept in touch with the girls and visited them often at medical school. They seemed to be enjoying themselves in a way that I never saw in any of the American medical students I met, and, what's more, they were beautiful women. I discovered there were guys in their medical class as well, but that a lot of the students were female.

During this time, I did meet a typical, blond Danish *shiksa*, and, after playing around in the back of my car a few times, she came to my room. I fumbled with the condom. She had no more experience than I, so the result of our fumbling and consequent consummation for the first time in a darkened room left much to be desired for both of us. But we both had fulfilled a mutual need to end our virginity. My landlady told me I had to leave the next day when she discovered the bloodstains on the sheets. It was probably not a moralistic gesture, but more a financial one—I had increased the cost of bedding, and she could not be sure that I would not do this again in the room. Dorte's sister, who had a serious boyfriend and was often at his place, said I could stay at her place until I left, which clearly was going to be soon after having received the pleading letter from my father. I wrote back that I did not want them to pay for a return flight, but that I would try to get a job on a ship so that I could bring the car home as well.

Puck walked the docks with me. At each ship I explained that I wanted to work on the ship, not for pay, but simply for my own transportation and that of my car. Each person I spoke to said they could not take me without seaman's papers. I went to the seaman's office and they told me I could not get papers without a job offer. At the Swedish tanker, the bearded boatswain asked me where I was from.

"New York—in fact, Brooklyn."

His eyes lit up. "I once had a girlfriend in Brooklyn. She was really something. We would get together whenever I came to New York. But that is over. I will give you a letter for the office, and, when you come back with your papers, I can take you. We sail in three days, but we start loading the ship tomorrow, so I need you then."

We ran back to the room, and I packed everything. I went to the apartment, said good-bye to the girls, and hugged each of them fondly. Lizbeth gave me a big passionate kiss, and I again thanked my lucky stars for the adventures this town had shared with me. I drove to the dock late that November afternoon. Peteris met me and told me he was from Latvia as he instructed me to call him Peter. He asked Lars, a Norwegian seaman, to show me to my room. There were four bunks in the room, two upper and two lower on each side. I was to have Lars, a good-natured, plump Dane, and a dark-haired Swede as roommates. Lars told me to park the car at the far side of the dock to be loaded the day we would leave.

The deck was busy the next day as loads of goods were directed deftly into the open holds. Lars seemed to be senior and well respected, often giving orders and, when there was a particularly tricky loading situation, he would take over the controls. As I watched a large crate of Tuborg beer being loaded into the hold, there seemed to be more jostling of the load than what I had seen earlier. As it came down, the corner of one of the net-engulfed crates slammed against the side of the hold and the crate broke open. I could hear yelling as the load was pulled up and over the side. The contents were quickly opened, the broken crate moved to the side, and the rest repacked into the net. The speed with which the broken crate of beer was removed made me realize that this must be the crew's ploy to sideline a supply of beer for their personal use without causing a fuss. After all, a few boxes of beer among the large numbers of crates would hardly be noticed. I marveled at their ingenuity and skill, not realizing that, later on in the trip, I would suffer as the target of some alcohol-induced denigration by the surly Swede about my role and position on the ship. Fortunately for me, Lars had taken a liking to me and served as a "protector," making sure that I was not taken advantage of or put in the way of harm.

I soon learned that the early December North Atlantic could be quite treacherous. Distant icebergs loomed huge on the horizon, even from miles away. When not chipping paint and performing other menial tasks, I was assigned a rotating watch schedule. Many of my shifts occurred late in the evening and lasted into the early hours of the morning. These periods of watch consisted of standing outside on the ship's bridge looking out for ships and icebergs while two senior crew, the captain, or one or two of the mates were in the wheelhouse, steering the ship and controlling the powerful and noisy engines.

Three days out from Gothenburg in Sweden, the sea and winds turned quite rough. I had a duffel coat, but, in order to stay warm, I wore all my sweaters underneath it. Fortunately, there were some raincoats onboard that I could wear over the coat; otherwise I would have been soaked by the waves crashing over the bow. At one point, I was told to go to the galley in the aft section of the ship and bring back coffee for the officers in the wheelhouse. The ship was heaving out of the sea in a noisy, rhythmic fashion. There was an unbelievable grinding of the propeller as it came partially out of the water when the ship rolled from side to side and from front to back. I was carrying the coffee in the dark, howling wind, holding on to the guide rope that stretched along the length of the ship when I realized that, if I went overboard, I would be lost forever, as no one would recognize my absence until the coffee, which I held in a stainless steel carafe in one hand as I groped and held the rope with the other, failed to arrive. I made it, received mild thanks from the captain, and returned to my spot on the bridge.

Within the closed portion of the bridge, I could hear the beeps from the radar getting louder. The first mate put his head outside and told me to keep my eyes open for the ship's sister, coming by from New York. Then, in the distance, through the fog and wind, I heard the sound of a ship's horn, first muffled but becoming louder as the beeps from within became closer together. As out of a dream, a ship with its lights on passed by at a distance which, to me, seemed almost close enough to touch. There was an exchange of fog horn blasts as we passed by each other quickly. I vaguely could see someone on the bridge of the other ship and waved, but our passing was so swift and eerie, I could not tell if my greeting was returned.

Five days later, the sun was up and New York loomed in the distance. We headed to the Brooklyn dock where, amid the crowds of longshoremen, I searched for my parents. I had sent them an express airmail letter telling them the name of the ship and the estimated date and time of arrival. The ship held me and the Renault. As we got closer, I scanned the shore in between my efforts to polish the brass fittings on the deck—the captain's attempt to spruce up the ship prior to docking. Then I saw them, bundled up for a late autumn day. I waved excitedly. They did not immediately recognize my bearded face, but then I saw my mother pointing to me, and they both waved. Three hours later, I was in the Renault, with its French license plate, hoping that I would not get ticketed before arriving home with my parents, who led the way in their white Chevrolet station wagon. I was home. Within an hour of entering the house and getting my backpack and small duffel bag into my room, unused for almost seven months, my mother said, "When are you going to shave your beard? You look like a rabbi." The next day, after showing it off to a few friends and neighbors, I shaved it off. Indeed, I was home.

I eagerly shared my travel experiences with my parents,

including my last weeks in Copenhagen—leaving out some of the more intimate stories—and told them that, if possible, I wanted to study medicine overseas. They listened, not quite digesting the implications of my announcement. I ended this first discussion with the notion that it would be a lot cheaper to study in Europe than in the United States. They murmured that they would consider anything, but, in the meanwhile, I would have to return to Brooklyn College for the spring term, a few weeks hence. That marked the beginning of a decision-making process that would change everything about my life. It came second only to the one I had taken some years before when, after having read A. J. Cronin's *The Citadel*, which completely turned my head around, I had decided to become a premedical student rather than pursue an engineering profession in my father's footsteps.

Was this decision based on my experiences with Puck, Dorte, and Lizbeth? I thought of my little tryst with Lizbeth and the loss of my virginity, unromantic and awkward as it had been, in the darkened rented room in Copenhagen. Or was it because of the laughter and glee I had experienced with them in their medical school classes that overseas study so magnetically beckoned? My being in Europe for those months had galvanized in me a desire to take a course different from that of my premedical friends at Brooklyn College. They all seemed to be looking for medical schools in the United States, becoming so fiercely competitive that they had a permanent sense of weight on their shoulders and seriousness in their hearts. I had seen a different world and wanted to experience the joy and freedom that seemed to be the norm in Copenhagen.

And so, on that day, I started to plan my strategy to get there—to Denmark, or as close to there as possible—one way or another.

Chapter 3

Dundee

Dundee was dark gray: the buildings all seemed gray, the sky was gray, and the first two days that I was there, it rained on and off the whole time. I arrived by bus from Glasgow, not realizing that the one I took was a "local"—it said Dundee on the front—and the conductress didn't think of telling me there was a faster bus as she muttered "Dundee," all the time cranking out tuppenny tickets in great numbers from her machine—finally giving me almost an arm's length of them. Dundee was ninety miles from Glasgow. Rain dripped through a crack in the window as the bus meandered in between and through towns and villages for the three-hour drive between the two cities. From time to time, I could see small houses through the rain-streaked window, especially when we got off the highway for a local stop, usually in front of a small shop that had a Players or McEwen's sign on the front with a packet of cigarettes or bottle of beer to illustrate the product. The driver sometimes delivered a package or picked one up, usually wrapped in brown paper tied with string.

I left my luggage at the Dundee bus station and walked around the city for a while, trying to get a sense of the city that would be my home for the next five years. The rain stopped.

I asked a local policeman about a place to stay and explained my situation—student, American, just off the bus, looking for a place tomorrow—and that I just wanted a place that would be not too expensive for overnight. He pointed me to a gray, three-story building with a sign over the entrance. It was a bed-and-breakfast, simple and, indeed, cheap. I brought my things from the bus station and walked up the two flights to my room. Later, dozing off, I could hear the rain starting again outside and awoke hungry.

My first Dundee meal was in a small restaurant near the bed-and-breakfast that the clerk had mentioned to me—also not too expensive—where most dishes on the menu were accompanied by side orders of toast, beans, and chips. (I had not yet figured out that chips were American French fries). I chose the fish and chips as it was a meal with which I was reasonably familiar. It was as greasy as anything I had ever eaten, but good and filling and, as I learned soon after, a staple in this city. Fish and chip shops were scattered all over the city, and the scuttlebutt was that the same oil had been used for years in each one of them. In those days, the meal came wrapped in newspaper that easily absorbed the grease. It would seep through the wrapper very quickly, leaving the diner by the end of the take-out meal—or takeaway, as the Scottish would call it—with finger-licking, greasy fingers. Those who did not like fish could choose another Scottish specialty such as white or black "pudding" made of meal and blood products cased in an animal-source intestinal cover. This particular delicacy sounded awful to me at first, but they actually tasted great. But they, too, were greasy.

I arranged to keep the room for another night and headed off to the university. Most of the buildings were close to the Perth Road and seemed very old. I wandered about and came upon an old, three-story, red stone building with Medical School written over the wide double doors that marked the entrance. I pushed and the door opened to a main hallway.

A staircase with a double wooden banister went up one side. On the walls were pictures of what appeared to be former professors, medical students, and athletes. An engraved brass information panel on one wall named the various departments and their floor location.

As I walked up the stairs, I kept thinking, *I left the United States to study medicine here? This building is ancient. This is the Middle Ages. What have I done?*

It will be okay, I reassured myself. *This must be the old building, and there is another one somewhere. Maybe this is just a museum.* I looked through a window in a door and saw a large lecture hall. Wooden seats ascended steeply. On the next floor were large glassed showcases filled with bottles of organs, each one carefully labeled—"Hashimoto's thyroiditis," "cirrhosis of the liver," "blocked coronary blood vessels"—with a small arrow pointing to something that I could not make out. There were hundreds of bottles of all sizes.

No one was around—the university was almost empty. I had arrived a few weeks early so that, after arranging for a place to live, I could go to Copenhagen for a week to visit my old friends. I found the registrar's office and met Miss Pierce, the woman with whom I had corresponded and who had sent me the telegram just a few weeks before offering me a place in second year. She told me that what I saw was, indeed, the medical school building and that most of my classes would be held there, with the rest in the various hospitals once I started my clinical work the following year. She clearly could read my face and said, "It is a fine medical school. Old building, yes, but fine people, you will see. It has a great history and tradition." I then asked where the housing office was located. She pointed out the door and said with a welcoming smile and rolling Scottish accent, "Great to have another Yank with us. We have had many wonderful students from over there over the years."

It was the third walk-up apartment—or, as I soon learned

to call it, "flat"—that I had seen. This one at least had an inside toilet, but was as dingy and dark as the two others I had previously viewed. When I returned to the housing office, the young volunteer said, "You are not going to find anything like what you might expect at home, especially not downtown near the university. The flats are old and none the best for wear, but students stay in them fine and you will have flat-mates as well. Sometimes a house comes up to share, but I have nothing listed right now. Maybe something will come up when the students return for the beginning of the month."

I did not want to wait or take a chance as I wanted to make my trip to Copenhagen. "Maybe something not quite in town might be a bit better?" I looked at the map of Dundee that she had behind her.

"Yes, there are some places, but they come with landladies and are not self-contained. A lot of students don't like that— they want to be on their own—you know, parties and the like." She gave me an address and showed me where it was— the Kingsway—across from the municipal golf course. "It is a bit of a walk—maybe half an hour—or a ten-minute bus ride. You don't have a car, do you? Some of the Yanks come with cars. Most of our students don't have cars."

I knocked on the door of the low bungalow, which was a few minutes walk from the bus stop where the careening double-decker bus had dropped me off. The conductress had pointed out the house for me when I showed her the address, and, when I got off, she'd said, "Cheery bye" so that it sounded like one word. I could hear a shuffling within and then the door opened, revealing a gray-haired woman in her sixties or so. "Hi! I'm Michael Gordon, the medical student the university housing office called you about." She invited me into a sitting room where heavy, floral-patterned chairs sat in front of a roaring coal fire.

"I'm Margaret Gilroy. I own the house. Tell me about yourself."

I gave her a short summary of my life as I looked around, taking in the knickknacks in the glass cases and the crocheted doilies under the little porcelain figurines and table lamps. There were a few scenic pictures on the wall and, over the fireplace, pictures of a couple and some young children. She showed me the house: three bedrooms, the sitting room with its fireplace and two overstuffed chairs, a dining room with a large table, and a kitchen with a smaller breakfast table. "This room is the one I am renting out," she said, opening a door. It had a double bed with a lovely wooden frame, a small table, wooden closet, and small dresser. "I put a hot water bottle in the bed at night and wake you up in the morning, if you give me the time the night before. Breakfast is a full Scottish breakfast, and you have afternoon tea and, on Sunday, high tea. If my son and his family are here, you can choose to join us for the lunch or have it on your own in the sitting room."

I could not believe my luck, especially when compared to the hovels I had seen earlier that day. "It is seven pounds a week," she said. I mentally performed a quick computation and realized that was less than twenty dollars a week—eighty dollars a month—a bit less than I had estimated for my rent alone, and here I was getting my main meals with it.

"Mrs. Gilroy, I would love to stay here with you, if you will have me." I was praying to myself.

"You know, Michael, I generally don't take students as they are usually too rowdy and drink a lot and come home late. I usually take young doctors, like Dr. Hunter, who is already staying with me—he's from Inverness … you know up the west coast. George is a pathologist so he has good hours, and he is very quiet, a nice, quiet chap. But you seem like a nice sort of lad, so I will have you here." I could not believe my good luck—a real house, a real room, a landlady to make me food, so I would not be on my own. I figured that, for my first year, this was the perfect arrangement.

She offered me some tea. The pot had a crocheted pink

cover over it that I admired and about which I commented. "We call them tea cozies. I love to make them when I am not knitting for my grandchildren." She picked up a blue swath of wool on two knitting needles, proud of her handiwork, saying, "For my three-year-old grandson." She looked at me as she handed me a plate and asked, "Biscuit?" which I soon learned was a cookie. "Michael, I was wondering what religion you are." I was stunned. I never expected such a question. I thought, and hoped, that this was not going to be some manifestation of anti-Semitism. My name was Scottish, and she certainly would not have known I was Jewish by the name—did I look that Jewish?

"Actually, I am Jewish," I answered in a manner I know contained a hint of hesitation and questioning.

Her face lit up and she said, "I thought so. As soon as I saw you through the door I said to myself, *Ach, another Dr. Shulman.* Do you know Dr. Shulman? He's from Glasgow. He was with me for two years. What a lad ... a real gentleman. I looked at you with your dark hair and eyes and thought, *Just like Dr. Shulman.* So I am extra happy to have you stay with me." I could not believe my ears as I abandoned my fearful thoughts about anti-Semitism and basked in her warm glow over my being Jewish—it was just too much. "Would you like some tea with your biscuit?" she asked. I put out my cup and, after she filled it, she asked, "Milk?"

I sat forward and said, "You know, at home we drink tea with lemon. I have never had it with milk, but sure, I'll try it."

She poured in some milk and said, "Doesn't it curdle—the lemon and the milk?"

"Oh no," I said, as I realized she had misunderstood me. "Not together with the milk—just the lemon; often with honey or sugar—the honey mostly when someone is sick with a cold." And then I added, with a chuckle, "Along with the chicken soup, of course!"

"I've never had it like that, but I have heard of it," she said. "They call it Russian tea in some places in town."

"Well, that's sort of where my grandparents come from," I continued amiably, "from near Russia, in what is now Lithuania." The time passed, and I knew I had made the right choice. That night, after I had brought over and put away my belongings, as I got into bed, I felt a warm, rock-solid object and realized it was the bed warmer, a crockery container filled with boiling hot water. The bed was quite warm, and, after the long journey, two days of travel and bed-and-breakfasts, and this day searching for a place to stay, I slept blissfully under the down cover, which weighed slightly heavily on me but welcomed me into sleep. As I drifted off, I knew I was in the right place.

I met George the next day and knew instantly that he would be someone who could help me figure things out. He was like a walking encyclopedia as he explained just about everything we talked about; the study of medicine for sure, but also travel routes and weather. He had a wonderful singing accent that I could understand, which I could not say for everyone I had met so far in Dundee. I left for Copenhagen the next day, visited my old friends—some of whom had served as my inspiration to come and study in Scotland—and shared some beer, stories, and laughter, but no sex (much to my disappointment), and returned to Dundee the day before classes were to begin.

I knew this world of Scottish medicine was a different one by the reactions of my professor and classmates to my tendency to raise my hand in class and ask questions. I was instructed that the goal of most medical students was to remain anonymous and, although I could not change my natural Brooklyn-bred inclinations, I toned them down. Some of my classmates learned that they, too, could ask questions without the world coming down on them. The year went by; in the summer my sister Diti visited, and, as I had promised when my parents said I could study in Scotland, we traveled Europe together—in a lime green Volkswagen. I had picked it up secondhand in Germany, where I had raced right after my last class. We used it to go as far south as Italy, ending our travels in Copenhagen where Diti met my Danish friends. That summer instilled a love of travel in her from which she has never recovered.

The next year's spring term, in 1963, marked the transition from the classroom to the hospital and real patients. I was becoming used to the accent, and hardly ever needed translation from one of my local classmates unless stuck for a word or a bit of slang. *Awa' wi ya*, meant "get lost," I learned, and so on. I would go to a pub after classes and have a beer with some of my classmates. They soon learned that one beer was my limit if they wanted me to stay awake. As a consequence, they were only too happy to treat me to a round from time to time, knowing it would just be the one and not go on and on as was the case with many of them, who drank amounts of beer I could never imagine consuming, and yet they suffered minimal side effects. They merely seemed to be a bit louder than usual, slightly tipsy perhaps, and assailed by an increasingly intermittent need to travel back and forth to visit the *loo*, which I soon learned was the washroom.

Following my clinical introduction before the second summer, I went home to work in a Brooklyn hospital. By this time, I had left Mrs. Gilroy's place and had lived in a few flats with various friends until I met up with Steve and we moved into the flat that belonged to Mrs. Dykes, right near the university. It was Mrs. Dykes, her dog, Judy, and the two of us—Steve, the dental student from London, and me, the Yank from Brooklyn. It was the spring term of third year in 1963, which was halfway through my second year in Dundee, that we began to rotate to different wards at different hospitals— lots of books and reading, putting the pathology together with the surgery and medicine, and trying to look like and act like a doctor on the wards, all the while eyeing the nurses or the female students (known colloquially and locally as "hens" and more generally as "birds") at the university. Medics, it seemed, had a reputation for being rowdy, bawdy, and, most of the time, inebriated. Since inebriation was not my forte, I aspired, at the very least, to discover just how bawdy I could be.

As the clinical years progressed and we came closer to being bona fide doctors, to our great pleasure we found that many of our classmates would seek us out to ask questions about their health. In terms of my aspirations, I found that practicing physical diagnosis on friends—especially female friends—was fun and sometimes a good way of "getting together." It was a grown-up form of "doctor," the game many of us had played when we were children. Unfortunately, sometimes this new physician's zeal would interfere in my relationships with women. Occasionally, I would become so entranced by the anatomical and physiological aspects of the sexual organs of a girlfriend that I would lose some of the romantic zest and focus, instead, on the appearance of her breast or vagina rather than seeking out its sexual function. One time in particular, I can recall percussing the rather lovely bare chest of an arts student, as if my hands were drumsticks—dum tee dum!—and she the drum, all the while explaining to her the different sounds, quite forgetting the sexual purpose of the initial groping and act of undressing.

One of the best parts of being a medical student came when we were told we could visit the emergency room at will, for it was only at this point that our involvement with actual patients began. Friday night was definitely the best time to visit *casualty* as the emergency room was called—in some ways, a more befitting term considering what we often saw there—and especially after the pubs closed on a payday Friday when workers had money in their pockets and a thirst in their throats. The good citizens of Dundee, a city marred by the historical Scottish Protestant/Catholic divide, demonstrated a continuing propensity to "act out" religious wars just as the pubs were closing and the guests were well intoxicated. Usually it only took someone yelling out, "Up the Pope!" or "Fuck the Pope!" that instigated a rumble that then became, much as in Leonard Bernstein's *West Side Story*, an all-out fight, with broken beer bottles and chairs as the weapons of choice.

They started rolling in about ten thirty or so, since the pubs closed at ten o'clock at night. The final call for drinks just prior to ten usually resulted in the *punters* (bar patrons) buying all they were allowed at one time, then quaffing the final pints of beers as fast as they could before closing time. This practice guaranteed them a state of severe inebriation, often to the point of coma and complete anesthesia. The latter was wonderful for us eager medical students. As the bloodied scalps, faces, and limbs were identified and any major bleeding stopped by the casualty officer and senior nurse, the drunks would be put behind a curtain and one of us assigned to "stitch them up."

I practiced my stitching at home all the time. I recall that, as a Boy Scout, I loved making knots and actually got the Scout merit badge for knot making. So here, with fine black silk or catgut suture material, I could oppose the ends of a cut quickly, make the knot so that it held, and then cut the ends close so my stitches would not unravel. I received some stitch instruction from older house officers whom I came to know during my various rotations and came to relish the "stitch it up" order. The scalp was often matted with blood, and the hair may not have been washed for a few days, though one would never know with all the blood around. A nurse usually cut the hair and sometimes shaved the area a bit so that the laceration was well exposed for the task of stitching. Sometimes last week's stitches were still in place, and we would just take out the ones from the past week before putting in the new set. Even though the normal protocol or best practice included injecting the site with local anesthetic, we knew that often the patient's state of inebriation had reached such an extent that nothing would be felt, with or without the use of lidocaine.

A night in casualty always ended with a fish-and-chip dinner from one of the late-night stands where young lads, ten and twelve years old, would be hanging around begging cigarettes off the customers. Some of them already had the telltale yellow fingers from smoking "fags"—the local colloquial word for cigarette—down to the very ends, whether filtered or not.

By fifth, and then sixth year, when it was felt that we had had sufficient clinical experience, medical students could take on *locums* (short for *locum tenens*), which meant filling in for a house officer who was on vacation. It was considered an honor and a plum job because the staff really got to know you. That helped if you really wanted to do well in exams, which did not seem to matter to many of my classmates, but mattered to me with my type-A personality and Jewish-Brooklyn background. My first locum was in the cardiology department, where they also looked after the patients undergoing new cardiac surgery procedures that were just being put into practice. Medical students loved cardiology because we got to use our stethoscopes, and understanding the mysteries unleashed through the magic of listening through those tubes was a sign of the erudite and enviable position of the "doctor." We all struggled with the sounds, but, when it happened, as it sometimes did, that what we heard was what we were actually supposed to hear, the epiphany was just too much of a thrill to let go. Much as kindergarteners do, we had to learn to share the experience with whoever was around to listen. The first time I heard the low-grade diastolic "rumble" of mitral stenosis, I knew I had mastered auscultation. You have to adjust your hearing to catch it, and, because of my musical training, figuring out when in the heartbeat it was occurring—systole or diastole—was the easier part for me. I could mimic the sounds quite well with my voice and then even "play" them on my stethoscope later on in my teaching career, rubbing my fingers over the diaphragm to demonstrate the heart sounds and murmurs to students.

Mitral stenosis is the narrowing of the heart valves from previous rheumatic fever—usually in childhood—complicated by rheumatic heart disease. The condition was still rampant in the 1960s in Scotland, especially in poorer towns like Dundee. We had been told by our professor to look for cases everywhere—on the bus, in the shops, on the street—as the telltale facial flush over the cheekbones and pinched features, often accompanied by difficulty in ordinary breathing in those whose valve was very narrow, were obvious in many of the citizens. In casualty, one of the real medical emergencies was pulmonary edema (fluid on the lungs) in a person with mitral stenosis. The patient would go into atrial fibrillation (very rapid irregular heart rhythm) as the narrow valve prevented the blood from being pumped fast enough. Patients would come into the department literally drowning in their own fluid and, if not treated rapidly, could die right in front of you. The only tricks in our medical bag in those days were digitalis, to control the heart rate, which took many minutes, if not longer, to work; morphine, to ease the shortness of breath and readjust the way the body handled the fluid; and bloodletting, whereby a large bore needle was put into a vein and a quantity of blood removed to ease the pressure on the stressed heart valve. These were the days before nice and neat plastic cannulas (small tubes especially designed to go into and safely remain in blood vessels with their exposed end available to take blood samples), so this last intervention was sometimes messy since blood gushed into a container from a straight wide bore needle in the arm, which was attached to some makeshift rubber tubing as the patient sat upright in bed fighting for life and breath.

Two dramatic things happened during this period of my

life when, as part of the locum, I would be in the hospital at all hours of day and night to learn. The first was witnessing my first open-heart surgery to repair a rheumatically narrowed mitral valve. This technique had come into being about a decade before I saw the procedure. It consisted of the surgeon making a small incision in the left atrium of the heart (the smaller of the two types of heart chambers) while the heart was pumping, putting his fingers or some sort of reverse pliers through the tightened, scarred valve, then pushing the fingers or pliers apart, thereby "splitting" the valve and increasing the size of the opening. When it worked, it was dramatic, with the patient waking up from the anesthetic clearly breathing easier and, soon after, demonstrating an increase in exercise ability. More sophisticated methods were developed years later to repair the afflicted valve, but seeing what was, in essence, the beginnings of open-heart surgery before the advent of the bypass pump was a monumental experience for me.

The second medical development during that period, which forever changed the face of heart failure treatment, was the introduction of furosemide, the first intravenous, injectable, fast-acting diuretic. I was on call with the house officer on "medicine." I was already finding that I loved medicine but had not started thinking about career choices yet. Medicine was always exciting—not in the same way as surgery, with which there was the drama of deciding to operate or not, and then the action of the OR—but medicine had all those stories which I loved—and the ensuing challenge of unraveling the story.

We were called to casualty where a thirty-something-year-old woman in pulmonary edema was struggling for air, her chest full of gurgling sounds, a sure indication of severe fluid accumulation. The heart rate was very fast, and digitalis had been given to slow it, but this reversal had not yet happened. The stethoscope revealed the irregular rhythm and low rumbling sounds typical of an abnormal heart valve due to rheumatic heart disease. The junior registrar came down, opened a small glass ampoule, and filled a syringe with the fluid it contained. The house officer who was with us wrote down in a black-covered notebook the name and age of the patient and what time the fluid had been administered intravenously. Eagerly, I listened to the chest, which was full of gurgling sounds (known in medical terms as *rales*), and explained to the two supervising house officers what I was hearing.

Usually by this time, preparations would be made for the bloodletting routine while waiting for the digitalis and morphine she had also been given to start working (which often took many minutes or more). As I listened to the chest, the gurgling sounds diminished very rapidly, and, within a very short time—which the house officer noted in the book— the patient looked up and said, "That's much better!" as she pushed the oxygen mask to the side. Shortly after, she asked for a bed pan and we could hear the gushing of her urination as she filled it, doing so again twenty minutes later, by which time her lungs were completely clear of *rales*. This was my introduction to a drug that would change the world of heart disease and which, over the decades, has become one of the staples in the treatment of heart failure the world over. In fact, I had seen the drug work before it was officially released on the market; we had been part of a clinical trial. Throughout the rest of my training, and in my practice since that time, I have used that lifesaving drug furosemide hundreds of times.

When I think about that first experience and my initial response to walking up the stairs in the old medical school building of Dundee, I realize that the telegram offering me a place was the best piece of good fortune that could have befallen me. My years in Dundee had such a profound effect on the shape of my life and my medical career that now, just the sound of a Scottish accent or bagpipe—even the sight of a piece of Scottish shortbread—brings a smile to my face and a sense of warmth to my heart.

*   *   *

She was on the other side of the High Street in Dundee, walking with two girlfriends. Her blond hair was bright in the sun on this unusually bright Dundee autumn day. As I passed her, I looked around and could see her look back for a moment in my direction. She continued to speak to her friends.

It was the fall of 1963, the fourth year of medical school out of the six-year curriculum, my third year in Dundee. (I had started in second year because of the credit they gave me for my premed university courses at Brooklyn College.) I had completed my first rotations of clinical medicine the previous spring. I had recently returned from a summer working in a hospital in Brooklyn where I went to visit my family and to hone some of my basic clinical skills. There I finally had been exposed on a daily basis to the world of illness and suffering and what, at the time, I felt were the miracles of medicine. Back at home in Brooklyn, I had engaged in an amorous relationship with the only female intern in the program. This gender imbalance seemed a bit surprising as, by the time I was studying in Scotland, a third of the medical class was female, a statistic that rendered the social aspects of a medical education far more interesting than what I saw to be the case in the United States during that summer visit.

Over the next week, I passed the girl I had noticed on the street a few times; I eventually found out that she was a first-year social studies student, and her name was Jeane. I was dying to meet her but did not know anyone who knew her well enough to make an introduction. When I saw her in the student union, the place was so busy and full of noise, I did not feel comfortable just barging in on her table of friends. At the time, the culture of the student union was such that, during lunch, most students sat and ate their light lunches with their own classmates or the few friends they might have made from other classes or faculties. I was still sitting primarily with the "medics" although I had a couple of friends in the engineering faculty, a predominantly male bastion in Dundee.

One day while walking down a Dundee side street, having just purchased a record in the only good music shop in town where I might buy a classical album, I literally bumped into Jeane, who was coming out of an adjoining knit shop. "Oh, excuse me," I said as I wondered whether I should just walk around her or get up my courage and finally introduce myself to her. As she moved her parcel of what appeared to be knitting supplies from one hand to the other, I went for broke and impetuously said, "I have actually wanted to meet you. I'm Michael Gordon, a medic from the States. I've seen you walking and thought we should meet. Do you have time for a coffee?" I was burning inside as I waited for what I anticipated would be some sort of rejection. Despite everyone thinking of me as very sociable, I was actually rather shy when it came to meeting women, and usually needed some sort of "situation" to get into the necessary conversation required to make the first move. I had always relied on humor to make my connections and, once started, could carry along well enough. I was just not good at getting things started. The direct approach I had just taken seemed far too blatant for me; I was sure it would bomb, and that would be the end of my quest for this green-eyed girl whose face, slightly red at the cheeks, I simply could not get enough of.

"Sure," she replied. "That would be very nice. I knew your name already—Linda, Ian's friend, mentioned it to me." As the heat rose under my sweater, I realized that she had inquired about me through a classmate. I could not believe it—she knew who I was!

"How about the shop down the lane? They have coffee and things," I suggested. As we sat down, I lay the recording of the Bach collection of accompanied piano music that I had purchased on the extra seat at the table.

"Do you like music?" she asked as she tentatively picked up the brown paper parcel that held the record.

"I do, and use it to help me study. These recordings from Czechoslovakia are really very good and very cheap. We do not have them in America—you know, all that communist stuff—and the Czech and Russian musicians are really great."

We ordered two coffees and scones, a Scottish pastry that I loved to eat with butter and jam—a great treat. I could not believe that I was sitting with this girl who was physically beautiful and exuberant in manner, and whose Scottish-accented voice was sweet music to my ears. "Where are you from?" I asked, trying to make out the region of Scotland she came from as she clearly did not have the Dundee accent, which was quite dense. (The Dundee accent was related in part to the commonly found, high-frequency hearing loss experienced by generations of Dundee women who worked in the jute mills. I recalled visiting a mill as part of my industrial medicine course to see the women who were not wearing their ear protectors because they said they could not hear each other above the unbelievable din of the mill when they were in place.)

"Troon, near Prestwick," was the reply. "On the west coast, south of Glasgow—do you know it?"

"I think I passed it once on a trip to Ayr to visit the home of Robbie Burns. Would that be right?"

"Probably so, but the town is easy to miss. I still make my home there with my parents and brother. He's in his next-to-last year of school, getting his highers next year."

"What's that, highers?"

"His last examinations to qualify for university. In England they have "A levels," which are about the same."

"I keep forgetting you go to university and medical school right out of high school," I said. "We need a university degree to go to medical school back home. That is how they let me into second year here; I already had three years of university."

"Home is where?" she asked, delving further into the mystery of my background.

"Brooklyn, New York; a place in the city called Brighton Beach."

"Aha! I knew you were a Yank by your accent, but I could not tell where in the States. I hope to go there—or to Canada—after I finish studying. I want to be a social worker."

Jeane, as she reminded me the first few times we met, spelled her name with one *n* and one *e* at the end—the only person by that name I have ever met who did so—and she said it with pride, "Jeane with one *n* and one *e* at the end." She would become the focus of my romantic and sexual life for almost three years, and in many ways represented much of the best of my years in Dundee. From her I learned about passion and restraint, sensuality and humorous abandon, and how Scots could consume so much alcohol without much of an impact; that is, if they were blond, green-eyed, and from the west coast. The Dundee of the sixties was still pretty straitlaced; there were no real drugs other than alcohol, which was treated more like an essential nutrient and lubricant for all social activities than the inebriant that it was. Birth control, which mostly meant the rhythm method, was often upset by the effects of alcohol, giving rise to a high birth rate among young girls whose weddings occurred not long before delivery and whose parents frequently adopted their offspring, which led to complex family relationships where mothers became siblings to their children.

Condoms were not readily available in pharmacies, at least not without asking the person behind the counter who, if a young lass, served as the best counterincentive to birth control efforts. Even if you got up the courage to ask for some *safes* as they were called, and the person was a male, his glare alone could be enough to counter any attempt at purchase. It was during my first visit to the barber that I discovered the prevailing method of procuring the means to avoid knocking up a girlfriend. The haircut complete, the barber removed the protective cloak from over me, shook it out, and, brushing the hair off my back, asked in his broad Dundee accent, "Will there be anything else, sir?"

I looked at him as I started to fumble in my pocket for the money to pay for my haircut and replied, "I don't think so."

He repeated again, with a wink this time as he looked to a box on the counter, "You're sure there's not anything else, sir?" He winked again at me quite deliberately. "The weekend is coming up, sir." I then realized that there were packages of condoms in the box and, feeling the blood rushing to my head, I shook my head, gave him the money with a tip, and left, hearing a laugh as I left. At least I knew now where family planning for students took place in Dundee. What I didn't know was whether or not you had to get a haircut to buy condoms, or if the barbershop was just one of the venues to purchase them. To be honest, I hadn't had much experience with them at this point of my life ... another lapse in my sexual experience and education. The first and last time I had used one had been on my first trip to Copenhagen, and that had been a bit of a circus.

Before meeting Jeane, I had already learned that much of the sexual activity between students was similar to what I had experienced in Copenhagen with Lizbeth and would probably be classified later on as "heavy petting," a combination of mutual masturbation and making many of the right movements, but always fully or partially clothed. It was a bit messier for the guys, but it satisfied most needs and certainly prevented conception, which, at that time before the onslaught of the more common contemporary sexually transmitted diseases, was the main concern. For sure, gonorrhea and syphilis existed in Scotland, but it was not something you would usually see, other than in really seedy folks or people officially or unofficially in the sex trade, whether professionals or really fervent amateurs.

So with Jeane, it would be three years of preserving her virginity while enjoying the most sensual relationship I had ever had before, and probably have had ever since. For the first year, during which we gradually and eventually gave up going out with others and became "a couple," she lived in West Park, the women's residence up the Perth Road. It was about a mile from my four-flight, walk-up flat in Airlie Terrace that I shared with Steve, Mrs. Dykes, and Judy the dog. For some of my time in Dundee, I had access to one sort of car or another. The first one was the lime green Volkswagen with German registration, which I had bought in Germany for my travels with Diti. Unfortunately, I had to get rid of it after the year that I had it in Britain was up. The second was an unmitigated disaster: an old Austin A7, purchased jointly by Steve and myself. It never had a working battery, so we would park at the top of Airlie Terrace and let it run down the hill, engaging the clutch as we reached the bottom, a technique that usually started the engine. We would be fine until we parked and had to start up the car again. If we could not park on a hill, there was the hand crank, which usually caught after two or three turns—and we were always lucky we didn't get a backlash, which could have broken a thumb. The doors were held closed by a rope across the front seat; but it ran— and that was enough for us—and only cost fifty pounds split between the two of us.

The problem with West Park was that it was closed to visitors after ten o'clock at night. Like many of the West Park girls' boyfriends, I became adept at getting in and out of the residence through windows and side doors at all hours of the night, despite the risk of being caught, which could result in expulsion. Jeane was on the ground floor, which meant my leaving—often quite late at night—could be accomplished quickly and with relatively little danger by a jump from the window should the door prove not accessible. The jump often resulted in a thud on the soft garden, but at least not a cracked bone.

As the year that we met progressed, Jeane and I started seeing each other quite often, though my routine stayed the same: study first, play later. I did not hang out much in the pubs after classes like many of my classmates. Instead, I ate a supper at the university or in one of the local cafes, which usually consisted of something with beans and tea and bread and butter with never a glimmer of anything close to green or fresh or raw on the plate. Afterwards, I would go to my room, put on one of my Supraphon records, turn off the lights, and go to sleep for an hour. Then I'd hit the books for another two or three hours, and, if pre-arranged, would fetch Jeane at around 9:30 or 10:00 PM. The pubs closed at ten, and Mrs. Dykes was at home most nights except for her bridge nights when she returned by 11:00. So we had relatively short periods of time in which to play—either in the flat at Airlie Terrace when Mrs. Dykes was out playing bridge, or in the car, which was fine until the weather turned cold. Then all we had was West Park with its relative comforts and serious risks.

After some necking and sexual rummaging around in the flat, and then in the car a few times, which included the embarrassment of almost not getting it restarted in the woods where we had parked, we decided to try our luck at Jeane's residence. By this time, Jeane had learned that many of the senior girls had their boyfriends there all the time with no bother, so we decided to try it ourselves. I would arrive at 9:00 PM. We would sit on her bed and talk about my plans, either for the next university break when I always went traveling to the European continent—the main reason I chose to study overseas—or for after medical school. Or we would talk of her desire to be a social worker and perhaps travel to Canada. We talked books as well, for we were both readers. Around 9:50 PM, we could hear doors opening and closing as people left, saying their good nights. Sometimes there might be whispers for a while longer, but, shortly after 10:00, with the curfew in effect, the place became very quiet.

The first time we were alone in her room, we just lay next to each other fully clothed, something we could not do in the car so it was quite a nice change. This night was the first time I knew for sure I had given her an orgasm—even though we didn't undress. As we moved against each other, her skirt lifting up so that only her panties separated us—me on top of her and her legs around my waist—I could not believe the strength of her arms around my back and neck. She opened my shirt so that she could massage my back with her hands as she grabbed me. After kissing me fervently, she lay with me and laughed about the probability of my being caught and sent back to New York.

"What would your father say about us, Michael?" She already knew that I was Jewish. As a Scottish Presbyterian who had met very few Jews in her life, she found me a bit of a curiosity. Once while we were rhythmically moving together, my Jewish Star of David fell forward; she let it rest on her face and then fingered it and looked at it. "Do you think your parents would approve of you being with me, a Christian?" I mumbled that it would not bother them as the rhythmic pace increased. I could not keep myself from smiling at the same time, marveling at her sensuality and the fact that here I was with this beautiful Scottish blond *shiksa*, the dream of every Jewish boy in Brooklyn. And she had just had an orgasm with me, and me with her, and it wasn't a dream, and my pants were sticky inside but I did not care. Later, I slipped out the side door around 11:30 with no problem at all—and even got the car going with just one crank. When I got home, I wanted to tell Steve, but he was asleep. This was the beginning of three years of passion, arguments, and sensuous making-up sessions.

"I do not want to lose my virginity until my wedding night," she had told me early in our relationship.

I do not want to make her pregnant and have to get married, because I am not ready for any of that, I repeated over and over to myself, aching with longing for her. Finally, one West Park night a few weeks later, a sequence of caresses through her underwear led me to move the fabric aside so I might feel, and then taste, her lovely wetness. This culminated in my bringing her to the point of climax, where I knew she wanted to go. She was reluctant to reciprocate the first few times, but, when she finally did, I could not believe the softness of her lips and my resulting explosion ... and what seemed to be her surprise when it happened. I had studied it all in physiology and anatomy, but had to admit that the theory and the reality were worlds apart. Even when I studied obstetrics and gynecology, there was virtually no focus on human sexuality—as if doctors would somehow understand it all as part of their inherent knowledge and experience—which I came to appreciate years after as false.

Oral sex would fill the void as we spent two years preserving her virginity, studied, made friends, broke up, and got back together, always with fervor and ever more questions about our future, whether that be together or separate. I met her family—kind, upright, solid, Scottish Presbyterians through and through. They were both heavy smokers, but it was the days when little was known about smoking and its adverse effects. Years later, long after I broke up with Jeane, I found their house again while touring the west coast on a visit to Scotland, and there they were, clearly quite ill and frail, with the effects of years of smoking showing in their pursed lips while they breathed and spoke. Jeane's father had a very barrel-shaped chest, and her mother's face was deeply lined. As if by coincidence, Jeane happened to call while I was there and they passed me the phone to say hello. She was far away in place and time—in Canada—where she had planned to go the last time we were together, just before I left to do my house job in Aberdeen and from where I went to Israel some months before the Six-Day War. I, too, lived in Canada by this time, but in a different city, and we did not talk about "getting together." She thanked me for visiting her parents; her voice had a lovely sameness to it.

During my final years of medical school and coincidental years with Jeane, I matured and began to understand there was an inner imperative driving me that I needed to explore alone before I could settle into a family situation. But sometimes, when we would walk the green fields or heather-covered hills together, I could imagine leaving my roots and my Jewishness behind to be with her, living in Scotland with her and raising a family so I might always feel her mouth on mine or her body moving sensuously and passionately under and over me. I would regain perspective during my trips abroad during the holidays as I met new people—sometimes other women—and realized that I was not ready to settle down; that, in fact, I had lots to do before that time would come, so that coming back to Jeane was always both a source of distress and great joy.

One weekend, we went to visit Chuck, my best friend from Brooklyn College days, who was studying for a year in Edinburgh after he finished his Navy service. We checked into a hotel under false names, which the clerk clearly recognized as such, asking rather obviously with a smile, "Is that Mr. and Mrs.?" I mumbled yes, and thus, we were "wed" on the spot. After the night out with Chuck and his girlfriend, we came back to the room—it was the first time we had been in a hotel room together—where the bedcovers had been pulled back to expose "satin" sheets. Jeane started undressing, first pulling off her sweater and then brassiere as she spoke to me. "I love you, you know, Michael."

I was stunned. I had not heard these words from a girlfriend since my last day in Brooklyn with Fran, the girl I left to pursue my studies in Britain. Fran had desperately clung to me and told me she loved me as she moved my hand to her crotch, something she had never done while we dated for almost a year. I remember pulling down her panties and being shocked to find dark pubic hair, which did not jibe with what I had thought was her natural light brown/blond beautiful mane. I became so fixated on the darkness of it all, that I pulled her panties back on and murmured something about my parents being too close by. I left her the next day when I flew to Glasgow and saw her again only once two years later on the street during a summer visit home to Brooklyn.

I did not know how to answer Jeane. I was afraid that, if I echoed her words, it would tie me to her for life, a problem I have had to contend with many times in my later years—and I was simply not ready for that. I did not know how to reciprocate words of love without implying a lifelong commitment. "You are so very beautiful, standing there with nothing on," I said, finally. She looked at me as I got up to hug her, my shirt rubbing against her bare breasts. She turned from me and went to the bathroom. I got undressed and slipped into the bed. "Jeane! Come to me. These sheets are something else! I want to hold you. Come!" I could hear the faucet in the sink running and then stopping, and she came out wearing her panties but nothing on top. She slipped under the covers next to me. "You can slide off the bed with these sheets if you're not careful," I said as she picked up the pillow and put it playfully—but perhaps with a hidden meaning— over my face.

"You might be shoved off the bed if you're not careful. Sometimes I really do not understand you." But then she sat up and threw herself on top of me. For the first time we lay naked together, no longer worrying that a matron might knock on the door or there might be a raid during which I would have to scoot out the window half dressed (which actually happened to a classmate of mine, and almost resulted in his being booted out of medical school). Keeping to our rule about virginity, we made "almost love," accepting that whatever we did with our mouths and hands was officially okay. When we checked out in the morning, a different clerk, who did not even look at our name on the invoice, was on duty. Remembering how we had called ourselves John and Mary, we laughed all the way back to Dundee.

During vacations, I traveled as planned, working in hospitals in each city I chose to visit. In Londonderry, Ireland, I had a bit of a dalliance with a local nurse from Donegal County who took me to visit her home, a small, three-room hut that sheep seemed to walk through at will. Her mother knitted almost an entire, complexly cabled sweater as we sat and drank tea.

I was short on my midwifery quota at this point in my career, so, when I arrived at the hospital in Londonderry, I ambled into the maternity unit, introduced myself to Sister (the head nurse), and three hours later had delivered the three babies I needed to complete my list. Delivering babies seemed to be a booming business there! I spent much of Friday night in emergency pulling fish bones out of tonsils and throats, and in surgery actually assisting at operations that I could only observe from a distance in Dundee.

Chuck joined me in Londonderry for my last few days. From there, we drove south to Dublin, having visited the tomb of W. B. Yeats on the west coast where Chuck, the poet that he was, recited some of Yeats's poems over the tomb, the wind blowing over the two of us. We slept in a bed-and-breakfast where there were crucifixes in every room and one in every stairwell. In the morning, we filled up on great amounts of toast, rashers of bacon, and eggs, and knocked back what seemed to be gallons of tea. Before we returned to Scotland and another year of studies, we pub crawled in Dublin with the locals and joined the groups in the inebriation, loud songs, and rude remarks that are the hallmark of students.

Our studies now moved into the hospitals, with clinical

rotations, long nights on duty, and locums, where I replaced the house officer and felt like a "real" doctor. I broke up with Jeane, but was as jealous as could be when I saw her in a pub one night with an engineering student. Though we had agreed to date others, once again we ended up in each other's arms. I helped her paint a new flat she'd moved into, but I became upset when she chose as part of her painting outfit the pink cashmere sweater that I had given her as a birthday gift.

"What do you care what I wear?" she yelled. "It's mine, you know. Just because you gave it to me doesn't mean you own it—or me!" Angrily, she pulled it off right then and there, paint roller in her hand. "Here, take it back if you don't think I know how to take care of it!" I ran to grab her, but she would not have any part of my advance. I left the sweater on the table, turning back to say good-bye as she stood in her bra in the middle of the living room. I ached.

The final spring 1966 term had come to an end. I had been accepted to Aberdeen for my house job. I would be returning home for about ten days to visit my family and obtain official government permission to stay overseas for another year, rather than doing my military service. Each year while at medical school, I had applied for and received the extension, so I assumed it would not be a problem. It was early June in 1966; I would be starting in Aberdeen on August 1. Jeane and I walked in the hills not far from where she lived. We lay on the grass, kissing and saying how much we would miss each other.

"This is really an important step for us," I said, "me, starting my house job, and you going to Canada for your social work certificate. We'll have to see what happens to each of us."

"Michael," replied Jeane, "I think you will start your traveling and forget about me and Scotland. I'm not even sure if I will come back home. I hear that Canada is wonderful … huge and with endless opportunities—who knows? My parents really want me to go."

I looked at her, breathing the sweet smell of her neck as I nuzzled her. "I could never forget you or Scotland. No matter where I go, I will always feel something special about this place. And you—no matter what happens to me—you will always be in my heart." It was the closest I had ever come to telling her how much I loved her, even though I knew, or at least felt at the time, that I could not marry her. As always, I was unable to separate feelings that were truly genuine from the ever-constant reality checking that was part of my personality.

We went back to her house. There was a note from her parents saying they would be away for the afternoon. "I'm going to take a bath," she said. "That was quite a walk we had, and I need to clean off." I could hear the water running in the old big tub in which I had bathed some time ago on one of my visits when we had stayed in separate rooms, all night. I lay on her bed, waiting for her to come out. She was wrapped in a towel, her long blond hair held up by another, turban-style, to dry it. She lay down next to me, and I pulled off my shirt and pants. I moved down to the inside of her legs and started to kiss her, anticipating the familiar rhythm that would follow as she spread them apart for me.

"Michael. Please make love to me. This will probably be our last time together."

Astonished, I looked at her and said, "I always thought you wanted to keep your virginity."

She laughed, "For what? For whom? I have to lose it with you, for if not you, who ever could it be? Please, love me and be gentle."

I pulled off her towel and slipped off my underwear. I was afraid of hurting her. I did not really know much about virginity other than the myths I had heard and that one experience on my first trip abroad many years before with a girl whose name I could no longer remember. I remembered groping in the dark under the bed for the condom I had put there and how, not having much experience, I had struggled to put it on with one hand. I had anxiously lunged into her, hardly feeling anything, yet, in my eagerness I came too quickly. Then, in the morning, I had seen the blood on the sheets.

But this was Jeane, the woman I loved more than anyone I had ever loved, even though not enough to wed her. This was Jeane, with whom I had shared every sensuous mode of making love short of intercourse. This was Jeane asking me to take away her virginity. It was afternoon; the room was lit with natural light. And, as I asked her if I was hurting her, she raised her legs. "I don't want to hurt you."

"It's okay, just go slowly." I could feel the little give as I entered and then, that warm, moist feeling. I was overwhelmed, and my head reeled. Again I asked if I was hurting her. She said nothing but just moved below me. I was afraid of the pleasure and suddenly felt fear. "Jeane, I don't have a condom. I am afraid I might come in you and I cannot help myself."

"It's okay, I'm about to have my period. It's safe. I knew this would be safe," she said in short breaths of heavier breathing. Then she stopped speaking, and I could not hold myself any longer.

"Michael. Thank you. It had to be you; no matter what happens to us, it had to be you." Enfolding her in my arms, I kissed her. I felt I had not been much of a lover; it had been too fast ... much too fast. "I wish I could have lasted longer, but it was too much for me. Maybe we can try again later."

"Shh, it was fine; this was it, my love. My parents will be home soon, and I need to clean up. And I need to wash the towel I put under me."

I looked down and it was red ... not heavily red, but red just the same. I got up and got dressed. Jeane put on a dressing gown.

Twenty minutes later we were having tea with her parents.

I left that night for Glasgow to take the overseas plane to New York.

Chapter 4

Eastern Europe—The First Time

Something was definitely wrong. I was feeling depressed, or down in the dumps at the very least, but it had been going on for far too long a time. It was the late spring of 1964, the end of my third year in Dundee, which was year four of the medical school curriculum. We had finished our first complete year of rotations in clinical medicine. As my low mood continued, each time I read about some serious disease, I wondered if my symptoms might be related to the particular ailment I was studying. Intellectually, I knew that it was common for medical students to have such experiences, but my questions felt very valid to me.

I started ruminating about death, associating terrible, chronic, debilitating diseases such as Crohn's disease or cancer with my own ultimate death. I had already taken the introduction to psychiatry course and liked the professor—Professor Greenblatt—whom I assumed, by the name, was Jewish. I tried to arrange to see him for advice, but, unfortunately, just as I inquired, I learned he was going to be away for a month. Instead, an appointment was made for me with one of the internists who taught us clinical methods. I liked him from his lectures, but I was not sure what help he could provide. I had already written to my best friend Chuck, who, after three years in the Navy, was going to do a post-graduate year studying English literature in Edinburgh. In my letter, I asked him a sobering question—if I were seriously ill with no hope of recovery, could I count on him to euthanize me? I could sense the groan in his letter as he responded, "Please, Michael, I love you dearly; don't ever ask me to do that."

"But, Chuck, who else could I count on? Only you!"

"Michael, I really hope you will never have to ask something like that of me. I think you should speak to someone."

"Okay," I responded, which is how I came to see Dr. Logan.

His office was warm and inviting, and the wood-paneled walls displayed a few nice pictures of old Dundee. His Littman stethoscope—the very latest in stethoscope technology … sleek and light—fit nicely in the pocket of his starched white coat. His Scottish accent was soft and mellifluous, unlike the harsh accent of working-class Dundonians to which I had become accustomed.

"You are from the States, aren't you? I recall you from the clinical methods tutorials last semester. Your accent sounds like New York—is that it?" He put me quite at ease, and, after a few words about my New York roots, he continued, "My grandfather helped build the Brooklyn Bridge. Lots of Scots went over and worked and came back with a good deal of money. He was one of them. I have pictures of him on the bridge. Quite an experience for a young man from Dundee."

After we had exhausted his Brooklyn connection, I told Dr. Logan that I was feeling quite "down" but did not go into the details about my death ideations, feeling somewhat uncomfortable revealing such seemingly absurd feelings to someone who might be teaching me again. After about fifteen minutes, he got up and put his hand on my shoulder, "You know, it is not all that surprising to feel the way you do. You are away from home and your family. Being homesick is quite natural. I am sure it will be okay. Write lots of letters, which you tell me you do. Keep it up."

I left his office realizing that he had not understood at all what I had been trying to tell him. The last thing I felt was homesick: I was exactly where I wanted to be and I loved my freedom and the opportunity to travel. Although I loved my family, I for sure did not "miss" them. Throughout my life, when I have spent time away from people who clearly love me as much as I love them, I have not "missed" them. Even in my later years, after I had established a family of my own, if we were separated by travel, this feeling of detachment or present-centeredness would be there. And, though it may seem cold and unloving, it is the way I have always responded to absence.

I decided to just focus on my studies. I had lost interest in the things that normally were very satisfying for me—food and female company. Music was still something I liked to listen to, but it often brought up morbid thoughts so I had to be careful what pieces I played. I actually lost weight—something that had never really happened to me before—and broke up with Jeane after telling her I just was not interested in seeing her—that I had to focus on my studies. It just seemed too much effort to go into the details, and I was going away for the summer. It seemed like a good idea to take a break from each other. I slept badly, ate poorly, but focused on my studies and tried to plan ahead. I had started looking into a summer in Poland as a travel and study opportunity and had already written to the students' organization to arrange the trip. Interestingly enough, though relatively unattached to the people in my present life, I wanted to get as close to my eastern European roots as possible, but there were no rotations in Lithuania or Russia, so Poland was as close as I could get.

The letter arrived confirming a placement in the Children's Hospital in Warsaw that would begin the first week in July. This gave me a couple of weeks from the end of term to travel there. While I was happy about it, I could not feel all that excited because of my miserable mood that would not lift. Although I could enjoy some company, it was limited. Having a drink—never a big activity in my life—just made me feel worse, so I avoided even the one beer that I often enjoyed with my classmates on a Friday night. The term was coming to a close. I was *swotting* (cramming) for my exams, especially pathology, as it was key to the following year's courses. I had a microscope that I had purchased the year before, and, in addition to the text, poured over the box of sample slides that I had borrowed from the department. I worked with them so much that, after a while, the red and blue images of the H&E stains (hematoxylin and eosin stains) filled my brain and began to look alike. I sat in the exam room as in a trance, writing away furiously. The bell rang. I was finished.

My bags were packed, and that afternoon Steve and I drove down to London in his red Mini Minor, dangerously passing slower cars in the A1's middle passing lane. I bought a Polish self-teach phrase book and tried to master a few terms. I knew that working with kids would likely be easier than working with adults, but thought that a few key phrases might ease the way. I had never really heard Polish spoken when I was growing up, and some of the phonetic spellings were quite a mouthful.

On the ferry crossing from Denmark to Sweden, I met a couple of female Danish students who were also on their way to Poland. They were quite taken with my ability to speak some Danish (which I had studied in Copenhagen during my half-year abroad prior to leaving for medical school in Dundee). We were together for two days, and, after months of numbness to female companionship, I began to feel an interest awakening in me. Finally, I was experiencing sexual thoughts again ... thoughts I had not entertained for a long time. Other than some handholding and a few kisses, there were no real opportunities, but the sense of optimism and fun was returning to me. By the time we reached Gdynia in Poland, where I said good-bye to them, I felt as if a darkened veil had been lifted from me.

I waited for the train to Warsaw with a few other medical students who were going there. We had a few minutes before it arrived, so I decided to go to the washroom before getting on the train, having experienced less-than-inviting washrooms on trains before. I walked into the men's room, and, while I was standing at the urinal, a fellow came and stood next to me. While pretending to pee, he said in broken, but clearly understandable, English, "Dollars, deutschmarks, francs, pounds. Anything you have—best prices—one hundred zloty to the dollar." Having just changed ten dollars at twenty-five zloty to the dollar, I knew this was a great deal. But it was the black market. I was very nervous: what if he was an undercover agent? This was a communist country. I asked almost foolishly, "Is this safe?" He looked at me as he mockingly zipped up his pants—"very safe"—and pulled out a huge roll of bills with foreign currency on the outside and zloty (which I could now recognize from my recent purchase at the exchange kiosk) on the inside. I furtively looked around the washroom and took out a ten dollar bill that I had in my pocket. Within a blink, I had a thousand zloty in my hand—ten one-hundred-zloty notes. He left saying, "Do vidzenia." I walked out a few moments after him wondering if the police would pounce on me. I could see him a hundred yards away speaking to some other students, with the wad of bills in his hand. The train whistled and I boarded for the last part of the journey to Warsaw.

*   *   *

The student residence on Karalkova Street was big. I checked in and found myself in a room with Peter, a medical student from Helsinki, Finland, who had been in the country already and was working on a surgical ward at the general hospital.

"The women are great!" was one of the first things he said after we introduced ourselves. "This residence is full of them— all medical students—unbelievable, dying to meet foreigners." It was not the first thing on my agenda, but I didn't mind his comments. Later that day, when we went out for something to eat and drink, I noticed a collection of attractive women staring at us as we went through the front door.

"You can have any one of them you like for a pack of chewing gum."

I had not realized at the time how coveted and expensive American chewing gum was in Poland. I thought of the nylon stockings I had brought with me on the advice of a fellow student who had spent some time the year before in Cracow. "You can get laid for a pair of stockings in that country—and for two pair you can shack up for a week," he had instructed me. I had immediately gone into Marks and Spencer's and bought a dozen pairs of panty hose, thinking that they would make me even more desirable. As a young man intent on experiencing the sexual dimension of life, this seemed like a reasonable gift to make to someone in such a poor country. It did not occur to me, then, as it would to the man I have become today, that I might have been taking advantage of their poverty and restricted access to Western goods in order to have my sexual needs satisfied. At the time, it did not seem particularly strange or exploitive.

The open-air cafe was full of students drinking beer and smoking and talking. A fellow came over and asked about foreign currency. I brushed him off and told Peter about my transaction at the border. He laughed and told me he had done the same.

He said, "A hundred is good. Sometimes you can get a hundred and ten, but there isn't much to buy here—food is just the basics. Good alcohol is hard to come by, and the beer is pretty pissy. They line up for good soap at the supermarket, but what most people end up using, which you can buy at a corner kiosk, is what we would call laundry soap. Not great, but it works. They don't even have coffee—there is some stuff that is brown and warm and has milk in it made from chicory root that is the morning drink. You get used to it, but what I wouldn't give for a good cup of coffee … even instant would be great."

The next morning I walked to the Children's Hospital with Geoff, a classmate from Dundee, who also had a room at the student residency. We had met the previous evening coming into the building. The *mleczko* shop (milk product shop) was across the road, and we each ordered the warm, brown drink that Peter had described. It wasn't awful, as long as it had enough sugar in it, but it was definitely not coffee. Of course, for a Scot to whom coffee meant Nescafe, it did not seem like a huge loss to Geoff. I had become used to tea over the years in Dundee, so I, too, did not feel the lack of that coffee aroma and caffeine jolt as a big loss. We entered the large doors of the hospital, and I showed my orientation papers to the clerk who was sitting behind the window just inside the door. She pointed up the stairs and gestured to the right. We entered the ward and found the head doctor's office.

"Welcome to Warsaw," she said in quite clear, if accented, English.

"*Dzien Dobri*," I replied, using the greeting from the first page of my phrase book. "*Jak si Pani ma?*" I continued with a standard phrase-book greeting, hoping I got the pronunciation correct. Geoff seemed quite impressed as the doctor's face lit up with a smile, and she answered in Polish. At this point I told her that I only knew a few phrases but wanted to learn as much as possible.

"*Dobze, Dobze*," which I indicated to Geoff meant "good"—so we were off to a good, friendly start.

As we were shown the ward, the youngsters laughed and grabbed and touched us as the doctor explained who we were. Some yelled, "America good" or "Thank you" as we passed, indicating their desire to connect to us. We entered the staff lounge, a small room with a table and a large teapot. Staff members asked if we wanted *herbata* (which I recognized from my phrase book as tea), and then introduced us to the other doctors, all of whom were women except for one older man, who spoke in clearly enunciated English, saying, "Welcome to Poland and to Warsaw and to the Children's Hospital. We hope you have an enjoyable visit." He introduced himself as Professor Berman, and I wondered about his name and roots. I knew of the massive killings of Jews in Poland and of the concentration camps, but did not know if there were any Jews left. And even if he were Jewish, he would not likely connect my name, Gordon, with my Jewish heritage.

*   *   *

Janos was twelve years old and from rural Poland. His heart was so big that you could see it beating through his chest. "*Cor bovinum*," the doctor said, and I recalled the term from my pathology book, never having seen a case in Scotland. "*Disease rheumatica*," she continued, and I realized she was talking about rheumatic heart disease, something I had already seen in Scotland, but in young and middle-aged adults, not pre-adolescent children. "Many times rheumatic fever, no antibiotics in village, no doctor. Very bad valves. Heart failure—take digitalis—very sick." Janos was very sweet and stuck his chest out so I could palpate it, heaving away under my arm. I listened with my stethoscope; the murmurs were so loud that I could not separate them or figure clearly from which valve they came. I put the earpieces over Janos's ears; he listened and smiled and thanked me with *"Dobze, tak."* I knew that Janos's prognosis was very poor. Heart surgery was still in its early days, and, from what I could see, would not be an option in Poland where, as I learned later that day, they still re-sharpened lumbar puncture and venipuncture needles rather than using the disposables that had only recently reached Scotland after having been available for some years in the United States.

The days were full on the wards, and my Polish was improving. After a week, I met a young Polish doctor who was doing advanced studies at the Anatomy Institute, and he invited me to meet some friends. The five of us met a few nights later at a cafe. All of them spoke English well. They told jokes, most of which had Russians as the butt of their humorous punch lines. They all wanted to go to England or America for further education; it was almost an obsession. "Medicine in Russia is primitive," one of them told me. "All new advances are from America or England. We get used journals and textbooks from there to read—and cannot believe difference in treatments." We began to hang out together in the evenings and sometimes on weekends. Sometimes others joined the group, including a very attractive but quiet woman, Wanda, who seemed to be involved with Bogdan, one of the students who was always talking about finding a way to go abroad. Bogdan's mother was a surgeon, and he wanted both of them to go away to study and maybe to live. Whenever I saw Wanda with Bogdan, she would look at me and smile a lot, but not say that much. Over time, I found that her English was quite good, and she loved to read English-language novels.

One day at the cafe, Andrej, another member of the group, announced that they had booked a sailboat for the coming weekend and would be going to Mikowike in the Lake District. He looked at me and asked, "Do you know to and do you like sailing?" which I interpreted as meaning, "Would I like to join them?" I nodded an enthusiastic yes, and it was agreed that he would arrange the trip. The limited experience I had had with sailing was with Professor McPherson, my physiology lecturer, who was originally from New Zealand and had taken me out a few times on the Tay estuary. It had been cold and blustery both times, but he was a master sailor, actually having sailed from New Zealand to Scotland when he took up his medical school appointment. Other than leaning when he yelled for me to do so, jumping from side to side, and, for short calm periods, holding the tiller, I had not picked up that much sailing expertise but found it invigorating. A three-day-long weekend trip on a lake sounded very inviting. The bus from Warsaw was quite full as our destination was a holiday and vacation spot. It was also the weekend, but we had room for our gear and decided to buy the food in the town.

The boat, which seemed to be about twenty-five feet long and could sleep five people, was owned by the Anatomy Institute and was available to faculty and students. It was waiting in its dock. Andrej and Bogdan went off to buy supplies and returned with the largest, dark, heavy rye breads I had ever seen, a big tub of margarine—white rather than artificially colored yellow as was the practice in the States— tins of preserves, sardines, and another kind of tinned fish as well as some eggs. They said there wasn't any meat in the store but that didn't seem to be a big problem. They had supplies for making a fire and some pots and pans so we could make hot drinks. The size of the huge round breads alone indicated that, however simple, it would be quite a feast. We got into the boat and stored our gear and food, and then Andrej, Bogdan, Iwan, and Borys, the latter two also from the Anatomy Institute, sat on the sides of the boat, looked at me, and said, "So, to sail." I nodded and agreed with a "*tak*." They kept staring at me. Andjej then said, "Why you do not to sail?" At that point I realized that they had thought I knew how to sail and had misinterpreted my interest as actual knowledge or expertise, which, of course, I did not have.

"I have only sailed with others. I have never been in charge of sailing, and know very little about it. I know a bit about physics and vectors but not much about wind and sails," I explained, drawing some pictures with a pencil on the paper that covered the rye breads. They all understood the physics principles.

They looked at each other and laughed and said, "So we learn to sail. Where is wind?"

We figured out where the wind was coming from, looked at the map of the lake and waterways, and decided in which direction we wanted to go. Bogdan threw off the rope, and I agreed to take the tiller. Andrew pulled up the sail and pointed to the direction we wanted, which was right into the wind. We pointed to the left and decided to sail perpendicular to the wind, which was away from where we wanted to go, but at least we would be on the lake rather than at the dock. The boat took off and we were going quite fast—almost too fast for us. Andrew told me to pull into the wind a bit so we would slow down. Finally, the tipping angle of the boat became less severe as our speed diminished. After twenty minutes, we were well on the lake but going opposite to where we wanted to go. We turned around, making sure no one lost a head, and started going back almost directly to where we had begun by angling ourselves so that we moved more in the direction we wanted. After an hour and a half of crisscrossing back and forth, we got the hang of it and finally started moving in the direction we wanted as the dock drifted farther into the distance and the quiet of the lake with its gentle lapping sounds dominated our experience.

We rounded the curve of one of the many islands that sat in the lake and encountered another boat. The guys started yelling to the occupants as if they knew them—which turned out to be the case. It was another group of young doctors.

On the deck was Wanda, who waved and said some words as well. Standing barefoot on the deck, she looked ravishing in shorts and a short-sleeved top. She exchanged a few words with Bogdan, who answered and shrugged his shoulders, and then we parted. A few hours later, well into the afternoon, we pulled into the shore. I could not tell if it was a large island or the mainland, but there was room to pull the boat up and set up camp, which was simple. We spread our sleeping bags under the sky, made a large campfire, and opened up our cans and jars. We cut large slices of the most delicious rye bread I had ever eaten. The group tried to keep me in the conversation as much as they could, but now and again they drifted into Polish. I heard what it was like to live under communism, but they also highlighted the stark differences between Poland (which historically had always looked to the West for inspiration and especially so since its fall to communism) and Russia, which they said was just "backward" and quite "ruthless," although they admitted it had become somewhat less so in the past few years. They had all gone there for some studies and joked about the poor quality of Russian medicine, even compared to what existed in Poland, which they acknowledged was backward compared to what they read about the West. Each expressed a yearning to go to America, Canada, or Britain—in fact, just about anywhere in the Western World. Bogdan mentioned that he had applied for a visiting fellowship to London and was hoping for word soon.

We had three glorious days of sailing and became quite apt at tacking and getting where we wanted to go. We never felt hungry, and my Polish improved more than their English. I really tried, though we had a few good laughs at my pronunciation and syntax, but it was all in good fun. Bogdan mentioned England a few times and alluded to Wanda with whom clearly he had a relationship. That much became clear from how the others reacted when he mentioned her, but, since much of that talk was in Polish, I was outside of it. We returned to the town and took the late bus back to Warsaw, exhausted but happy with our trip.

Two days later, I met Wanda just outside the hospital. She was not there because she was studying pediatrics; she had come to deliver a package to one of her colleagues. We walked together a bit, and then I just asked her, "Would you go out with me for dinner tonight?"

She looked at me intently, her deep brown eyes glancing over my face. "Sure. I know a small restaurant that actually has some reasonable food. You know it is hard to get good food in Warsaw, but, because tourists go to this one, it is not bad."

"How about if I meet you at the tram crossing at the end of the street where you live—it is not far from me—at seven tonight?" Then I did something I had seen the Poles do. As we were about to depart, I took Wanda's hand and brought it to my mouth and kissed it. "*Do vidzenia*," I said, in my best pronunciation. She smiled and nodded her head as she turned to leave.

The meal was very simple: cabbage borscht, bread, and some sort of dumplings with potatoes, followed by what seemed to be a treat—an apple cake—with the make-believe coffee I was becoming quite used to. The one thing I noticed about it, which was a bit disconcerting, is that it gave me a lot of gas. The only saving grace was that, since everyone drank the stuff, gas production was quite universal!

We walked to a park, sat on a bench, and then walked some more as I took her hand, to which I felt no resistance. She told me her life story and how her parents had survived the war in a smaller city, Czestochowa, in the south of the country. She said she was a small girl when the Nazis were defeated and the city liberated by the Russians early on in 1945. As we talked, our hands entwining more, I revealed that I was Jewish, even though I was a student from Scotland, and told her of my Lithuanian roots. She turned and looked at me intently, "You know that all the Jews were killed by the Nazis in my town during the war. There was a big community; the synagogues were destroyed, but the Jewish cemetery is still there." Her eyes welled up in tears. "There are almost no Jews in the medical school now, almost none in Warsaw, but I have a friend whose mother is Jewish and she lives in Warsaw. And Professor Berger—the pediatrician—is Jewish. He is very famous, you know."

As we walked, she pointed to a somewhat run-down block of apartments and said, "This is where I live. Do you want to come up and visit?"

I felt my heart leap at the thought. "Yes, I would love to." I momentarily thought of Jeane in Dundee, but that seemed a long way off, and we had broken off with each other before my trip.

"I share the apartment with two other students, but they are both away so it is empty," she said as she unlocked the door. The place was small, but neat, with some nice pictures on the wall. "One of the girls collects art pictures. These are from a trip she was allowed to take to France some years ago—from the museum." She took me to the sitting room and said she would get something to drink. It was a diluted fruit drink—mostly sugar and water—but it was refreshing because it had been in the refrigerator, a small affair but in working order. The top button of her white blouse was open, and I could see the upper mounds of her breasts as we sat facing each other.

"Tell me," I hesitated. "Are you and Bogdan a couple?"

She turned away from me a bit and smiled. "We were, but I do not think so now." I leaned forward, and we kissed. "He likes his freedom and goes around with different women. He says they do not matter, but it is very hard for me." I pulled her closer and kissed her again as my hands moved to the front of her blouse and opened the next button, exposing her breasts even more. We were on her sofa, and easily moved from sitting to lying next to each other with her facing away from me, curled into me and my arms around her, my right hand moving into her blouse. I unbuttoned the rest of her blouse and helped her out of it. I started to move toward the clasp of her brassiere as I kissed the back of her neck. Her smell was very earthy and natural; she was not wearing any perfume.

Then I heard her sob, quiet at first and then louder. "Stop! Please let us just lie here." She leaned over and grabbed a blanket that was at the end of the sofa and pulled it over us. "I like you. You are so nice. I never imagined I could be with someone Jewish. I never thought what it could be like. But you are going away soon and that would be painful and I cannot stop thinking of Bogdan. I do not want to do this. I know he does this but I cannot. Is that okay? Can we just lie like this and talk and not have lovemaking together? I am sorry but I can't."

She continued to sob. I touched her face and kissed it, tasting the salt in the tears. "Yes, that is okay. I think you are a lovely, beautiful woman and would love to make love to you, but I would never want you to be sad or resent me. So let us just be like this and talk." She leaned over and turned the light off. She turned to face me, with a smile and kissed me gently, non-sexually and curled back into me, clearly relieved.

It was a strange experience for me, yet one that had happened before in my life and would happen again in the future with women to whom I was attracted, including the girl I was in love with throughout my adolescence. She loved me as a friend, while I was smitten with her all those years. We could curl up together quite often to talk, sometimes about her latest love or disappointment. I would lie there, just happy to be with her, suppressing my sexual urges so not to risk losing what we had. Years later, before I left for medical school in Scotland, we attended a summer school course together and had the preamble of an actual physical relationship. Kissing her had been a yearning for so many years that I could hardly contain my joy. We lay together and explored each other somewhat, but clearly sex was not forthcoming, especially in those days. We actually discussed the possibility of marriage and her coming to Dundee with me to study art. We talked and talked and then, suddenly, as if nothing had happened, she told me that she could not marry me or go to Dundee and would be going to Cornell. We hugged and I tearfully told her that maybe some years might have to pass before we connected again. Years later, during my internship in Aberdeen, I had a deep relationship with a Norwegian medical student, but she, too, wanted only a friendship having just recently lost her lover, killed the year before in an automobile accident. We would lie curled up together in front of the fireplace in her living room listening to Brahm's *Second Piano Concerto* as I yearned for her love but acquiesced to her deep friendship, hoping that one day she might change her mind, which she never did.

A few days later, Bogdan came to the pediatrics department looking for me.

"I have been accepted to a fellowship in London. I am leaving in a month. I will be there for six months. I will do research at the Hammersmith Hospital—you have heard of it, yes? I am very happy."

I congratulated him, as did the other staff members who were standing in the office discussing some cases.

"May I speak to you alone for a minute?" he indicated to me. We walked into another room. "I wonder if you can help me, as I know you come from Britain. The government will not let me take much foreign currency out, and I know I will need more than I can take. Is there any way, if I give you zloty here, that you could arrange for me to have money in London?"

I thought for a minute and wondered to myself if the

parents of Steve, my flatmate from medical school, could help. "I will see what I can do. How much do you need?"

"Maybe fifty pounds."

It was not a huge sum, but an amount that I could not imagine how to spend in Poland. But I thought, if this was the help that Bogdan needed, then I would try to provide it for him. I made the call that evening and, despite the poor connection, made the arrangement. I told Bogdan, and he asked me to come to his apartment the following evening so he could give me the zloty.

The apartment was small; he lived with his parents. His room was clearly one of a medical person, strewn with lots of medical books and some old medical journals that looked very well read. There were posters on the walls from European cities—Paris, London, Rome. "Sit down," he invited, pointing to a chair. He pulled a pile of zloty from the desk drawer. "You know the exchange rate is twenty-five zloty to the dollar. I will be giving you seventy-five, which is three times the rate. I hope that is okay with you," he said with a smile.

I briefly thought of saying that I could get one hundred to the dollar at any cafe, but decided that it would be impolite since he had been a good friend to me and perhaps did not know about black market rates. He likely thought he was giving me a very good exchange, and, for him, it was clearly very-hard-earned money.

"Thank you," I said as I took the money and started putting it into my pocket.

"No, please count it. I want you to be sure that it is the right amount."

"I really don't have to; I trust you," I replied. He then said some words in Polish and followed with, "That is an old Polish saying which means 'when doing a financial transaction, always act as if the person you are doing it with is a Jew.'"

I looked at him, speechless. He continued, "You understand that Jews are very shrewd with money and one has to be very careful and exact with them to avoid being cheated. Therefore, the saying."

"And do you believe that saying is accurate?" I asked.

"Well, I have to be honest; I have not really done any financial transactions with Jews. There are not many left in Poland, and one does not see much of them in business. A few of the doctors are half-Jewish, and the professor of pediatrics— that older man—he is Jewish."

I took a deep breath. "Bogdan, you have just had a financial transaction with a Jew. I am a Jew, and I trust that what you have given me is the amount you said you would, without my counting it. And the people who will give you the money in London are Jewish. And the reason they are doing this for *you* is that they trust *me* and know that I will give them the money when I return because I want to help you."

By this time his face was completely pale. He stood and started to say something.

"Please don't apologize," I said. "Just remember this event. Here is the name and phone number of the people in London you are to call. They are the parents of my best friend and will be very kind and generous to you. They will probably invite you to dinner, but you do not have to feel obligated. Good luck."

I shook his hand, turned, and went out the door. I was hurt and offended, but realized as I walked down the street from his house that what he had expressed was part of the collective anti-Semitic culture that had been part of the history of this country for centuries. I felt a mixture of anger and sadness and almost forgave him for his ignorance, but believed that someone with his education should have known better.

I finished my final two weeks in Poland, which included a short trip to Cracow that was full of student fun. I made contact with Professor Berman, and we shared some tea as he told me how he had survived the decimation of Polish Jewry by being a student in Switzerland during the war. After he returned, despite what had happened, he resolved to stay and help rebuild the country and the medical faculty, which he did as professor of pediatrics. He was now, in fact, retired but kept busy at the department. After meeting with him, I sought out the memorial to the Warsaw ghetto where so many Jews had perished. As I wandered the streets, I realized that, although my family had been from Lithuania and had left prior to the Second World War and the Holocaust, this world could very well have been theirs. They simply would have perished in Poland rather than in Lithuania, as did the remnants of their family in 1944 when they were shot outside their village. I realized that the world that was so full of Jews in Eastern Europe was no more, but the mythology about them continued to exist even among people who had hardly, if ever, met one.

I saw Wanda for a brief moment while I was arranging to leave and gave her a warm kiss good-bye, which she returned with a smile.

"Meeting you was very special," she said. "I will never forget what we shared. *Do vidzenia.*"

I gave her the package of stockings I had carried with me from England, which in fact had not lived up to the promise of my acquaintance who induced me to buy them. I knew that Wanda would be happy to have them and told her to not open the package until after I had left.

Not long after, I managed to get a spot on a boat going from Gdynia to Helsinki. My previous experience as a seaman when I had returned home from Denmark three years earlier, and the fact that I still had seaman's papers (which I always keep with me along with my passport), were enough to get me on board with room, board, and passage in exchange for work. A fair deal, in my estimation! It was a Finnish boat, and they recognized my seaman's book as Scandinavian, which was valid with them. After two days and two nights, I arrived in Finland with some gifts I'd bought with the proceeds of the exchange with Bogdan, including silver earrings with some typical green Polish stone which I had bought for Jeane, hoping we might rekindle our relationship despite the way it had ended before the summer. I ended up with many unspent zloty, since there was so little to buy of interest to me in that impoverished country.

My fur hat, which I purchased in a tourist gift shop before I left the country, would always be a warm reminder of that remarkable summer in Poland.

Chapter 5

Playing the Piano and How Music Helped Me Be

His name was Mr. Bergunker—at least that is how I addressed him even though I knew his first name was Max, the same as my father. It may have been changed when he arrived from his native country, which I always thought was Russia, years before I started taking piano lessons from him. I was six years old and had already developed the habit of banging out tunes on the Sohmer baby grand piano that filled the combined living room/ bedroom in our one-bedroom Brooklyn apartment.

Because of the housing shortage in the post–Second World War period, my family moved into my maternal grandmother's lovely Brighton Beach apartment on a "temporary" basis, which proved to span a dozen years or so. Grandmother, herself an immigrant at age fifteen from Lithuania, shared her small space with me, my sister, and my parents.

I shared the bedroom with my sister and my grandmother, known in our language as Bubby. The apartment had a lovely view of the beach and the ocean, and during all those years of sharing, I would hear the ebb and flow of the waves. From my grandmother, I heard stories. My love of stories probably is strongly related to those many nights when we lay in our beds with the lights off and Bubby told stories of her life. I have vivid images of pogroms, of Cossacks riding through her village brandishing their swords. My grandmother hid in the potato cellar only to emerge the next day to see death all around her. I could almost feel the undulations of the ship on which she traveled on her own as a fifteen-year-old from her native home in Eastern Europe to the golden shores of America. I could picture her working in a sweatshop in the women's garment industry, and I joined her in her raucous support of the International Ladies' Garment Workers' Union.

But it was her connection to music that bound us together most intensely. She had a beautiful voice and sang in a Yiddish choir. As I got older, she took me to some of the marvelous, massive performances of song and dance at the Yiddish theatre in Manhattan's old Jewish District on 2nd Avenue. I loved those magical outings with her, and we went often, just the two of us. We met friends from all over with whom she spoke either Yiddish or Russian or some other language besides English. She seemed to know so many. I once asked her how it was that she spoke so many languages. She replied, "Where I grew up, from day to day you did not know who was in charge, so the more you could speak, the safer you would be."

She could be very critical of those who *chose* to be ignorant, a state she differentiated from stupidity, for that was an inborn trait she felt a person could not help. The greatest two denigrating abuses that she would hurl at someone or mutter under her breath were "know-nothing" in English and *paskudniac* in Polish-Yiddish (which means a bad or lousy person).

I believe that it was my connection with Bubby that was ultimately responsible for my becoming a geriatrician. I had never thought about it, but now I recognize how often, when dealing with an older woman—especially a Jewish one from Eastern Europe—I feel a deep kinship that must have its roots in my childhood experiences with Bubby. Over the years I have adopted a number of such elderly patients, each of whom I have asked to be my honorary bubby, to which they invariably say yes with apparent happiness.

My mother was quite artistic. I knew she had danced ballet and modern interpretative dance when she was younger and was always recognized for her grace and rhythm, even when dancing at a family wedding. This talent continued even in her later years when she danced with seniors' groups at public performances or at her beloved senior center where she taught dance classes. She also played the piano. Her mother had purchased the Sohmer, which filled much of the living room space of the divided room, during the Depression for twenty-five cents a week. The embodiment of culture, it still remains in our family's possession, now in the home of Neta, my eldest daughter.

This exposure to music took many turns over my life's development. The weekly lessons with Mr. Bergunker were core to its development, even though I did not cherish the experiences or even always find them pleasurable at the time. By age seven, I was walking more than a mile to the piano lesson alone. As I plunked away, I experienced alternately warmth, wrath, compliments, or criticisms from the teacher from whom came utterances of joy or dismay in broken English depending on how diligently I had practiced that week. On the top of his upright baby grand piano, sitting in a silver ornate frame, was the calligraphic axiom, "Success is 1 percent inspiration and 99 percent perspiration." With this dictum looming just above eye level, I would know I was in trouble when Bergunker's long stick, with which he tapped out the timing and rhythm, would fall with a crack either close to my hands, on the keyboard, or, in moments of sheer exasperation, onto the furniture in the piano room as he threw it into the air. He would thwack the stick with great force and bluster as he questioned with a modest degree of spittle whether I had actually sat down and practiced as I had promised him the week before.

That was always a complex question to answer. In general, I was very good at the *sitting down* part of the practice routine. My mother worked out of the house some days a week. My grandmother was not responsible for my practicing and was often busy sewing in the next room, listening to the Yiddish radio or reading the *Jewish Daily Forward* (or *Forvitz* in Yiddish), which I dutifully bought for her every day from across the street at the candy store. I, for sure, would *sit* at the piano as I had promised my mother—and usually soon after I came home from school. There was a clock on the piano, and I was committed to practice an hour every day. When I was feeling less inspired—which was quite frequently depending on what book I was reading—I might move the hands on the clock (which had years before lost its glass face) a bit forward to make time move more quickly. The clock's enforced movement was gradual and incremental—and then, suddenly, it would be 4:00 PM! When my mother asked if I had practiced for the hour, I could say with a straight face—despite the increased pace of my heartbeat, which reminded me I was stretching the truth—that I started at 3:00 PM and had played until the clock read 4:00 PM. My mother, dear believing and loving soul that she was, never questioned the veracity of that statement, just as she never questioned the upset stomach or headache that I feigned years later when I hated my junior high school homeroom and English teacher and scored about thirty sick days in a nine-month school year.

But Bergunker liked me, and, despite my lack of total commitment, I progressed nicely and played each year at his annual recital. With time, he placed me later and later in the program along with the more advanced pupils. The bane of my musical existence at age eleven and twelve was Pam Strauss, who was in the same grade at school as I and the very paragon of musical virtue. She was perky and self-possessed, and her parents were also just too good for words. They would extol each and every one of her musical virtues at every conceivable opportunity. Deep down in my heart, I really could not stand her, but always managed to be gracious and would grovel before Pam and her parents. We often followed each other in the recital program, with Pam always playing after me as the hierarchy of accomplishment required. My mother confided that I had more feeling in my playing, but that Pam was a "technical wizard."

One year, Bergunker upended me completely. He proposed that Pam and I perform a duet for two pianos at the final recital and chose Saint-Saëns's *Carnival of the Animals* as our piece. I hated rehearsals because Pam was always perfect. Bergunker had placed the two pianos side by side in his small apartment studio, and I could see her to the side of me as we practiced. Her hands were perfectly held; mine, rather on the large side, tended to sag, something Bergunker constantly tried to rectify by carefully placing his long stick under them as I played. This usually resulted in my having to stop because the stick tickled. I would agree to try harder and hunch my shoulders to get into what was an unnatural position for me. Pam, of course, just played away flawlessly. Bergunker hardly had to speak to her other than tell her just how well she was doing, which elicited a smug smile from her as she glanced sideways at me. I was just beginning to become sexually aware and, as we practiced, would try not to stare at her burgeoning bosom, which was beginning to stretch the nicely starched blouses her mother always had her wear that, according to the fashion standards of the time, went perfectly with her plaid, pleated skirts.

At the final recital, I had two pieces to perform: the duet with Pam and Chopin's *Fantasy Impromptu*, which I had diligently learned and, according to my mother, had mastered.

Even Bergunker complimented me on my feeling and, for the most part, dexterity prior to the actual recital, which took place at Steinway Hall in Manhattan. It was a bit formidable as my parents, sister, grandmother, and I sat through the performances of the younger age groups, groping their way through their pieces. Then it was time for the duet. Pam was as prim as could be, in an ironed, tailored white blouse in which her just-budding breasts pushed forward under an almost, but not completely, concealing bra. The two pianos faced each other, which differed from the way we had practiced side by side. I could see her serious but composed face across the uplifted Steinway lids. Mr. Bergunker mouthed, "One, two, three," and we started. I was in a daze, but the music wafted across the two pianos into the audience as we rode the musical tide together, bringing more passion and feeling to the piece than we had ever done in practice. It was almost sensual the way we finished the final passage and chords together, and the audience applauded with enthusiasm. I both hated and loved Pam in that moment, for she seemed so composed throughout it all while I was exploding with inner feelings.

Then it was time for my Chopin. I felt all eyes on me, especially my mother's, which I engaged just before I adjusted the seat, wiped my perspiring hands, and started to play. I was floating along, feeling that I was sailing or flying when I came to the second part and then, suddenly, a blank. I could not find the correct notes to start. I could see Bergunker to the side. There was a pause in my heart and brain that seemed to last for an eternity. I paused for what seemed like another hour, then started the piece again from the beginning, hoping that I might surely find my way the second time, moving from one movement effortlessly to the other. As I came to it, I released control of my hands so they could move in a way that was almost disconnected from my brain. And then, suddenly, I was there, moving effortlessly through the second and then the final movement, playing with all the passion and feeling that I could muster. I finished. There was a moment's pause, and then applause that filled my ears. I could see a big smile on my mother's face as probably only she and Bergunker, who was also grinning broadly, really knew what had happened.

When we received the 33 1/3–rpm recording of the recital and listened to it, we could laugh at how it seemed that I had effortlessly restarted, adding two first movements to the piece and ending up with a flourish. Pam knew as well as I what had happened, but that did not bother me. She was the last student to demonstrate her skills on the program and, of course, played her piece flawlessly, though in my very biased opinion, without any real feeling. Years later, after I had left the neighborhood for medical studies, I was surprised and saddened to hear, despite my mixed feelings about Pam, that she had given up music, had not pursued a higher education, and seemed to be "in deep trouble" by my mother's account, the details of which were never explained to me.

In spite of these early challenges, music would become the key to my existence, and I used it throughout my life to help me deal with challenges and channel emotional feelings that might be troubling me. As I became more interested in female companionship and sex—even though in those years it was still a pretty taboo activity for single men and women, no matter their hormonal and emotional pressures and urges— music was one of the ways in which I connected to women. It was often almost a test of any level of possible compatibility and, amazing as this seems, would either take the place of what might be considered foreplay or its follow-up, which, in the limits of those days, would probably more accurately have been categorized as heavy petting and not "going all the way."

Two pieces of music are deeply imbedded in my psyche and always invoke great emotional response. One is Rachmaninoff's *Second Piano Concerto*, which I first heard in my home when I was about seven years old and my father brought home a 45-rpm record player that plugged into our old radio. With the player, he also brought a five-record set of the Concerto and its common companion piece, the *Rhapsody on the Theme of Paganini*, recorded in 1946 by Arthur Rubinstein with the NBC Symphony Orchestra. The records were red vinyl. I listened to them endlessly, anticipating the pause as the records dropped into place automatically and the arm holding the needle landed on the outside groove and quickly moved into the soundtrack.

Years later, after my grandmother had died and I shared the room only with my sister, I purchased my own 33 1/3–rpm turntable. Like the 45-rpm model it replaced, it, too, plugged into a radio. I went to Manhattan's Fifth Avenue record emporium, the Record Hunter, an icon of music stores, which later closed in 1992 after being in business for forty-seven years. There, I bought a newer 33 1/3–rpm version of the Rachmaninoff concerto. When it began playing, I couldn't understand the fluidity of the music, forgetting that the pauses I had become used to over so many years were no longer necessary as multiple records didn't have to "drop" for the music to continue. It took me many weeks to readjust to the new recording, whose music moved smoothly from movement to movement without artificial interruptions.

The second piece that speaks to my soul is Brahms's *Second Piano Concerto*, for it was that piece that connected me to Lisa Schnerer, a Norwegian medical student whom I first met on the ferry from Norway to England when I was returning from a holiday ski trip to Dundee for my medical studies. I was immediately attracted to her. She had long, blond hair, blue eyes, and a rather pointed, but straight, nose. Over the years we would run into each other from time to time and, although I expressed an interest in coming up to Aberdeen where she was studying one year behind me, she never followed through with a welcoming response. When I accepted a house job (internship) in Aberdeen, one of the many reasons was to pursue developing a deeper relationship with her. We met and visited and listened to music together, our favorite piece being the Brahms. I came to understand that she wanted me only as a friend, and I accepted that role while still hoping for something else. We would often lie in the dark together on the floor, on a blanket, my arms wrapped around her clothed body, listening to her copy of the record. Our relationship never went beyond friendship, and, even years later when we corresponded, often from very far away, it would always be as friends. When I hear the Brahms, I always think of Lisa and those winter nights on her floor with a fire burning in the fireplace and the music wafting across the two of us; me, yearning for her love, and she ... I will never really know.

Music helped get me through medical school. Good recordings of high quality and low cost were readily available from Czechoslovakia on the Supraphon label, which featured outstanding musicians unavailable in the United States because of the anti-communist fervor that still existed in the early 1960s. I tended to be a late-night studier. Once I had my own room and could buy a record player, I purchased a 33 1/3–rpm changer without the case and found a wooden box in a grocery store in which it sat nicely. I hooked it into an amplifier I had bought in a secondhand shop in Dundee, the site of the clinical campus of the University of St. Andrew's Medical School. My routine was to have supper, either at the university dining room or, in later years, in a shared kitchen dining area. I would then take a nap listening to classical music, which soothed me into slumber for an hour or two. On awakening, I would hit the books with music always playing in the background. The ability to study, read, or write with classical music as my companion has never left me.

I carried my record changer and amplifier with me wherever I moved, and it was one of the first things to be set up in a new room. The speakers were basic, but adequate to my needs: these were the days before reasonably priced earphones, so those living in the same flat or medical intern's residence with me often remarked on my musical tastes. I had few nonclassical albums. Music was always in my life during those medical school and postgraduate study days. In fact, my love and knowledge of music once probably kept me from an awful jam on the border between Bulgaria, where I had been visiting, and Greece, where I was going to work in an Athens hospital as a medical student

It was the summer of 1965. I was driving my car south to do a month in a Greek hospital followed by a month in an Israeli hospital, this being the first time I would visit that country. I had met Boris Teofilova, a Bulgarian émigré musical impresario in Munich where my friends Laszlo and Marlene lived. Laszlo, a Hungarian refugee from the 1956 revolution, and his Australian wife had invited Boris to dinner as part of an entertainment evening for me. He was very lively and almost a caricature of an impresario, with a wide, black handlebar moustache. When he heard about my planned trip through Hungary to visit Laszlo's family and thence on to Yugoslavia, Greece, and thereafter to Israel, he asked if I might consider going through Sophia, Bulgaria, where he had family, especially a niece who was, in his words, "a wonderful violinist." I looked at the map and saw that, after I went down the Yugoslavian coast, I could move inland through southern Yugoslavia and cross into Bulgaria not far from Sophia. Since I was always up for adventure, I decided to do it. He gave me his card and wrote the name and address of his niece on the back and a few words of introduction on the front. He said to just show the card to the family, and they would welcome me with open arms and great hospitality.

In Hungary, I spent a few days with Laszlo's family: his father, a regional family doctor; his wife, who ran his office and the household; and his sister, who worked in the wine region in Sárospatak in northern Hungary where they lived.

Laszlo's father took me on medical rounds to the Gypsy village where he was the doctor. As soon as he arrived, dozens of children gathered around chanting his name and holding his hands with glee. He had delivered every one of them. He could not speak much English, but, during house calls to some of his sick patients to whom I was introduced, he explained in a mixture of German, English, and Latin medical terminology what was wrong with them, the signs of which were often very evident to me—such as an older woman whose breast cancer had eroded through her skin and for whom only local dressings and pain medication were available for treatment.

The night before I left, Laszlo's father took me into the back garden, which was somewhat overgrown and, in a corner, put his hand into what seemed to be an old section of drainage pipe. He pulled out a wad of currency, all in western country denominations—dollars, deutschmarks, francs, and sterling—and handed them to me saying, "For Laszlo, okay?" I wasn't sure in that short moment how I would get the money to him, but assumed that, once I was out of Eastern Europe, I could find a way. I took the money, put it into an envelope, and secured it with a rubber band. I took off the underside of my VW Beetle's dashboard, which was held in place by a few screws, and hid the money there for reasons of safety. It was not an amount of money I wanted to carry around. I left the next morning to continue my journey through to Belgrade, where I secured my visitor's visa to Bulgaria.

The driving through the rough terrain of southern Yugoslavia was very slow and poor. Although roads appeared on the map, in reality they were often of very poor quality—gravel in places and broken asphalt in others. The large patches of remaining winter snow here and there did not make the journey any easier. I had picked up two male hitchhiking Swedish university students who were willing to bounce around in my VW Beetle to go just about anywhere for the adventure. When we were halfway through Yugoslavia, night fell, and, without lights, the road appeared to vanish just as we entered what appeared to be a small village. We could see light in a number of houses, and smoke coming out of chimneys. Having the confidence that came from many years of traveling in Europe, I parked the car, walked up to a house, and knocked on the door. A teenage boy opened the door with wide eyes as I said as quickly as I could—in all the languages I knew, "Do you speak English, French, Italian, Polish, and German?" The boy stepped back, and a young man appeared and said in broken, but intelligible, English, "I do. Who are you?" As I replied, I could see half a dozen people come to the door to take a look at me over the shoulders of the man. They all began speaking to each other in a Slavic tongue.

The two Swedish fellows were hanging behind me trying to figure out what was going on. The next moment, we were whisked into the house and the door was shut behind us. Everyone took our hands and shook them, and they patted us on the back. We entered a room where a big fire blazed. We were seated around a table. Very soon, soup and bread appeared as a woman who seemed to be our English speaker's mother busied herself in food preparation at a large cookstove. We stayed up quite late as the family gleefully showed us pictures of the young man who spoke English from his three years in the United States where he had visited and worked in construction—they were somewhat tattered black-and-white shots—but they told us his story of adventure and hard work in "Hamerica." The family provided us with beds and feather-filled comforters to sleep under as the rooms got quite cold during the night. They also showed us the location of the outhouse, which we all made sure to use before going to sleep to avoid risking an accident should the need arise later with everyone asleep and no lights on in the house. The next morning, they loaded us up with bread and cheese and some onions cut up into pieces and sent us on our way. Clearly we had brought great pleasure to the family, and they, in turn, had given us a wonderful experience.

The children ran after the car waving at us as we left. The way was really just the remnants of a road that had great gaping holes in it, lots of snow, and large rocks, which we had to try and avoid. Gradually the road became more passable, and, after many hours, we came across a sign in a number of languages, including English, pointing to Sophia, our final destination. We passed through the border with little difficulty and no suspicious interest in the contents of our car or the fact that the two hitchhikers and I had passports from different countries. We were waved on and made our way to Sophia, arriving at about ten in the evening. I found my way to the center of town, and there was the Grand Hotel in the middle of the town square. Since there did not seem to be any alternative, I asked the Swedes to wait in the car while I went to ask about a room. With the exchange at the time so favorable to the U.S. dollar, I assumed that, whatever the cost, if split between three of us, it would be reasonable. We would get our bearings in the morning and figure out future plans. For my part, I intended to go on alone to find the Teofilova family and leave the hitchhikers to make their way without me.

I entered the lobby to find it quite ornate but run-down, and went to the front desk. I asked about a room for three and showed the clerk my passport and visa. In broken English he asked, "You have a reservation?" When I shook my head no, he indicated that, without a reservation, it was impossible to provide a room. I explained our situation, and he shrugged and turned to some papers on his desk. I took out the card from Boris Teofilova and asked the clerk where the address he had written down might be. He looked up at me quizzically and said, "You know these people?"

"Her uncle is my friend," I replied.

He walked with me to the front of the hotel and pointed

to a dark, somewhat run-down building on the far side of the square from where the hotel was situated and said, "There." I drove the car, still carrying the two drowsy Swedes, over to the far side of the square and checked the address in the dark to make sure it matched the one on the card.

I walked up the stairs, on each floor pushing the hall light button, which let the lights on for about thirty seconds. I tried to read the names on the doors. They were in Cyrillic, which I had learned some years before when I had tried to learn Russian on my own, but gave up before I got very far. I got to one landing where the bulb was out, but had the flashlight from my car, which I turned on, and there was the name I was looking for which I spelled out to myself. It was 10:30 PM according to my watch. I knocked on the door. A few moments later, I could hear whispers through the door. The door opened a crack and the word "*Sto*," or something like it, came out. I could see an eye and part of a face. I quickly said in English that I had been given Irena's name by her Uncle Boris in Munich, and I slipped his card through the crack in the door. The door closed, and I could hear voices behind the door speaking rapidly in whispers. The door opened a crack again, and a woman's voice asked in English who I was. I replied quickly, but with as clear English as I could muster, "Are you Irena? I am a medical student from Scotland, and I met your Uncle Boris in Munich. He asked me to visit you if I came through Sophia, and here I am. Sorry it is so late, but the hotel would not take us in and I did not know where to go to find a place to stay. I know it is 10:30 at night, and I am sorry to disturb you." The door closed and then opened fully to reveal a thin, dark-haired woman in her mid twenties, an older man and woman behind her, and a teenage boy next to her. She ushered me in and closed the door quickly, "It is actually 11:30 at night here, and we were worried who might be knocking at our door at this time of night. Please sit down. Would you like some tea?"

I sat down and then realized the two Swedes were still in the car. I explained, and Irena's brother went down to beckon them up into the very small apartment. Within an hour they had fed us and had rearranged beds and rooms so we all had a place to sleep. The next morning, the Swedes went on their way after thanking everyone profusely; the trip had been quite an adventure for them. I stayed on for three days as Irena's guest. She played the violin for me and gave me gifts of her records that we could not hear as she did not have a working record player. While walking together in Sophia one afternoon, we passed a shop that sold Western-style electronic and household products. She said, "It is the store where you can buy goods for dollars. Only useful for those who have a source of western money from family or who work in the embassies or hotels where they get tips in foreign currency." I walked into the store, pulling her behind me by the arm, and went straight to the section where gramophones were displayed. There was a modestly priced, compact, self-contained, 33 1/3–rpm, Dual, German-made player with a built-in amplifier. I had just that amount of dollars in my wallet. I asked the assistant if we could hear it play, which she agreed to. The sound was lovely, so I took out my wallet and bought it immediately. That evening, we listened to Irena's recordings on the player, which I gave to her as a gift. In return, she gave me copies of the programs from the concerts where the recordings had been made, signing each of them in English with a large flourish—"Best wishes," or "Fondest regards," and her name.

Before leaving, I packed the two recordings of her music that she had given me and the many programs on which she signed her name. I left for Greece two days later, having learned all about her life and the oppression experienced by both Irena and her dear uncle whom I had met. His crime was having studied English literature in the United States. Hers was being connected to the West through her uncle in Munich.

"Most of the time they leave us alone," she told me. "Sometimes they bring us in to the police station for questioning. When I go abroad to travel, anywhere—even within the Soviet bloc—I have to get permission, and some of my family must always remain here."

After I had driven for about seven hours, the terrain became more barren and sparse and the road became quite narrow, but at least it was paved. The sun was low on the horizon as I entered what was clearly the border post that separated Bulgaria from Greece.

I stopped my car, and the policeman took my passport. He went into the small immigration and customs office, and I could hear him speaking to someone inside. A man wearing dark pants, a light-colored shirt, and dark glasses came out and asked me in broken, but understandable, English to get out of the car but leave the key inside. "Sit down, please," he ordered, pointing to a wooden chair with its back to the south as he pulled up another and turned it backwards while continuing to face me. I could see two policemen opening the doors and the front "trunk" of the car which, of course, in the VW was not the engine as that was in the back. They started taking out all my belongings, stacking them next to the car. I anxiously wondered what they might do or think should they remove the dashboard cover and find the foreign currency that Laszlo's father had given me. I assumed initially that it would just be confiscated. A frisson of terror ran through my body as I realized that they might think I was a smuggler.

"So, what were you doing in Bulgaria? I see you do not have a stamp in your passport of the hotel you stayed at. Where did you stay? All hotels must register visitors and stamp your passport."

I felt nauseated as I realized the predicament the Teofilova family and I might be in. "I stayed with family of a friend who is a Bulgarian music impresario who lives in Munich." I took his card out of my wallet, which fortunately, with the idea of letting him know we had connected, I had taken back from Irena after she let me into the apartment. He turned the card over and asked, "And how do you know him?" I looked around and saw that the place was desolate.

"I am a musician as well and know him through the music world. I play the piano." I had a nightmarish flash that they would take me to a piano and ask me to demonstrate my prowess.

"And who is this family you stayed with?"

"She is his niece and a well-known violinist in your country."

"You did not go to the police station to register that you were staying with a private family?"

"I am sorry, no. I did not realize I should, and maybe they just forgot. I arrived very late at night, and they were very eager to make me comfortable and then show me Sophia over the next two days."

I saw the policemen stop emptying the car—in any case, the ground contained everything that was in all its compartments—but they had not found the hidden money. One of them indicated with a few words and hand signals that there was nothing to be found.

"Tell me, what did you speak about for two days with this family?"

I could see the sun reflected in my interrogator's sunglasses and thought of the interrogation scenes in Koestler's novel *Darkness at Noon*. I realized that, if anything happened to me here at this desolate border outpost, no one would ever know. Stupidly, I had not contacted anyone in my family or any of my friends about my plans other than in the most general way, and even that had been weeks before, prior to my entering Eastern Europe. I looked directly at my interrogator's face, as I could not really see his eyes, and replied, "We talked about music. We listened to music. We visited the music school where she teaches and the symphony hall where she plays. Let me show you," I volunteered, pointing to the package I could see piled with my belongings on the ground. He took off his glasses and told one of the soldiers to bring the package to us.

"Here, you can see!" I pulled out and handed to him the two records and the half dozen concert and recital programs, all of which featured Irena as well as her greetings to me. He turned them over in his hands.

"Nothing else but music?" he questioned, looking straight in my eyes.

I looked back into his eyes, now no longer hidden since he had removed his glasses. "What else would we talk about?"

"Politics, maybe?"

I tried to hold myself steady and said, "I have no real interest in politics. Music is my passion, my love, and Irena shares that with me."

He motioned to the two policemen to put my belongings back in the car, which they did with great care. He went inside the office, stamped my passport, and returned it to me along with my musical package and Boris's card, though not before he had written down an address in Sophia. Finally he said, "If you ever come back, you must register with the police." He waved me on; the two policemen saluted me as they pulled up the barrier, and I drove past them and entered Greek territory. There, about fifty feet away, I was met on the other side by Greek border guards who stamped my passport, gave me some English-language tourist materials, and pointed to the road I asked them about.

I hoped that Irena and her family would be safe and thanked the heavens for the gift of music that had led me through this frightening situation. I laughed to myself at the thought of what I might have done if, suddenly, they had produced a piano from somewhere and asked me to play. I could probably have done justice to the *Fantasy Impromptu* even if I had to play the first movement twice!

Chapter 6
Aberdeen

They called to say that she was coming to ward four—the fever ward. "She is in her late twenties, very sick, high fever, delirious, with a rash covering her whole body." That was the message from Sister Douglas, the head nurse, who had got it from the referring family doctor. I was very nervous. It was my second day as a house officer at the Aberdeen City Hospital. I had finished my medical studies in Dundee just a few months previously. Here, patients were admitted directly to wards without the benefit of an emergency room triage and diagnosis. The two medical registrars were offsite, as was the chief of medicine, who was in charge of the unit. Prior to his recent move to Aberdeen, the chief had been one of my favorite professors in Dundee the year before. He had invited me to join him as a house officer, which, for me, was too great an honor to turn down.

I saw the ambulance stop in front of the one-story elongated hut, built as a temporary unit during the Second World War and still functioning as part of the hospital, now made up of a dozen of these buildings, each separated by fifty feet or so, and surrounded by grass and a few low-lying bushes. Within minutes the patient was on the bed, burning hot, her body covered with a fine, red rash. The sister came in with me as I examined her. The patient was mumbling, and her lips were dry and cracked.

"Sister, I can almost lift her whole body up from the bed by the back of her head, her neck is so stiff. What do you think? Meningitis?" I asked, looking intently at the patient as I ran my hands over the rest of her body, examining her chest, heart, and limbs. Sister nodded in agreement.

"I need to do a lumbar puncture, I think," I said, looking again at Sister Douglas, who had already signaled to a junior nurse to bring out the LP tray. Sister did not say much, and I had only met her the day before, but, as was usually the case with the sisters I met during my studying days in Dundee—sixty miles to the south—their wisdom and confidence was most often expressed in their actions, cool-headedness, wealth of experience, wisdom, and directedness.

"Sister," I said quietly, so that, if the patient were conscious enough she would not hear me, "I have done only one lumbar puncture and that was with supervision. I know the theory but have not had much experience."

"Not to worry, we're here to help," she said comfortingly as she started pulling the over-the-bed table to the side. Then she called in one of the staff nurses. "Get the patient positioned for the LP. Have her face the window with her back to the door side of the room," she directed to the rosy-faced, young staff nurse in the starched wide skirt and blue blouse standing by her side. The nurse rolled up her sleeves and put the LP tray on the table that was now by my side of the bed. She went to the other side of the bed and, with the help of another nurse, rolled the patient onto her side and curled into a C shape, the back of her hospital gown open to reveal the spinal vertebrae. The patient was thin, and I could see all the spinal processes, just as in the anatomy textbooks I had pored over during those early years of study in Dundee. I thought of the "fever hospital" in Dundee where, during one of my rotations, I had done my first and only LP, a senior doctor directing my hands, on an older man who was not deathly ill and for whom there was time to set things up slowly.

The staff nurse opened the tray cover in a sterile fashion, and I put my hands into the latex gloves—sterile, powdered, and tight fitting—that she held open for me as if I were a surgeon. I knew that, from now on, I could touch only what was on the tray and had to be very careful. Having put the surgical mask on before starting, I worried about the mist that began to cover my lenses as I breathed. Sister took them off my nose and coated them with a bit of lens cleaner she had in her pocket to stop the misting. A nurse poured iodine into the stainless steel kidney dish; I opened up and spread the folded gauze.

"Check the manometer and the fittings before you start," Sister said, "to be sure everything is working. Remember, you put in the needle until you feel the 'pop' and the fluid should come out when you remove the stylet from within the needle. As the fluid comes out, we collect some in each of those three test tubes on the tray. Then put the manometer on the needle and turn the handle for the pressure. Then we pull the needle and put pressure on the insertion site. Clear?"

I nodded, trying to hide my fear. The patient was very sick, and I knew the LP was crucial to making the diagnosis. Her neck was arched back a bit, typical from what I had read in books about meningitis. But I had never actually seen a new, fresh case; only a few patients, recovering some days following treatment. I wiped the spine with iodine and could see Sister nodding next to me. As I took the alcohol swab to clean off the iodine, I glanced up as she stood by, silently, with a look of approval and support. The patient's head was to my left and, with my right hand, I felt for the space between L4 and L5 spinal processes which were nicely stretched by the young nurse, who was keeping the patient in a curled position. All eyes were on my hands which, surprisingly to me, were not shaking as I first put in some local anesthetic, waited a few minutes, and then eased the long, new type of disposable LP needle in at an angle.

I felt the tissue's slight resistance as the needle moved forward and then the "pop" that told me I had passed through the layer of *dura mater* that surrounded and protected the cerebrospinal fluid and spinal cord. I carefully pulled out the stylet, praying inside myself that it was not a "bloody tap," which might occur if I had hit a blood vessel rather than making a clean piercing of the tissues into the spinal fluid space. The yellowish, turbid-looking fluid came out in a jet, indicating a clean tap, high pressure, and certain infection. I gathered the fluid into the three test tubes, put the stoppers on them, and gave them to Sister Douglas, who stood with a gentle, knowing smile on her face as I slipped on the manometer and measured a very high pressure. I pulled the needle out and applied pressure to the entry point. The second nurse took the tubes and said she would run to the lab, which I knew she meant literally as it was in one of the other nearby huts. The laboratory was waiting for the specimen as they had already been alerted to the case.

We turned the patient onto her back as the nurses cleared the tray and table and produced a couple of blood culture bottles and syringes. Sister said, "Remember, two sets, five minutes apart, in case you contaminate them." I was good at venipunctures, having spent a summer as a medical student in a Beth-El Hospital in Brooklyn as part of the blood sample team. I had done hundreds of them and knew I could get into almost any patient's veins. This patient was young and, although on the "dry" side because the fever had caused dehydration, presented no problem in securing the samples. Sister smiled at the two nurses and said, "Fine. Let's get the drip set up so, when the lab calls, we can decide on which antibiotic to start. I expect it will be penicillin as this rash looks very strep (short for the bacteria streptococcus) to me, but we'll wait."

The intravenous clear fluid was hanging, with a needle now in the vein (plastic cannulas—small tubes used for intravenous procedures that were becoming available in the United States—had not yet made it to Aberdeen City Hospital). I taped the needle in place and secured a board to her arm to prevent her from moving it. By the time I finished, the call had come through to Sister, who came in and said, "Streptococcus on gram stain. The cultures should be ready tomorrow afternoon and the penicillin is just about ready to go." I put the first small bottle of penicillin on the infusion pole. I took the needle hanging from the bottle's plastic tubing and plunged it into the yellow latex–topped "piggyback" port. This was a few inches from the end of the main tubing that led from the infusion bottle into the needle that I had earlier placed into the vein in her arm. The small bottle containing the penicillin emptied over fifteen minutes, and I visualized the bacteria being surrounded by the penicillin molecules, while leucocytes attacked them.

The phone rang down the hall, and the staff nurse called out, "It's Dr. Ross. He's about twenty minutes from the hospital. He wants to know if you need to speak to him before he gets here."

I put my head out the door and told the nurse, "Tell him we have a twenty-eight-year-old woman with streptococcal septicemia and meningitis who has been LPd and cultured and has just been started on IV penicillin."

The nurse called for Sister. I could hear her on the phone, "Fine, he did just fine. Good lad. He's a Yank, you know. See you soon, Dr. Ross."

I checked the IV—the fluid was running in quite fast—and we would just have to wait to see what would happen. I was sitting by the bed when Sister peered in the door. "Good job ... with a bit of luck she'll pull through." She went up the hall, leaving me alone with the patient. The staff nurse who had helped me position the patient came in to fix the bed and smiled at me.

Outside it was a mild August day, overcast but not raining. In the distance, I could hear the downshifting of gears and the whine of the engine of the older model sports car that was propelling Dr. Ross to the hospital as he maneuvered along the coast road that led to the hospital. He came into the room with the appearance of a controlled rush, pulling his white coat on. He looked at the chart and notes that I had carefully written. We had met briefly the day before as he did his orientation. He was only about two years older than I, but was four years ahead of me in training. He felt her pulse and lifted the back of her neck and said, "The heart rate is coming down, and she sure is stiff. Good job!" For the first time in my life, I felt that I was a doctor.

The fever ward was not limited to adults, a somewhat strange arrangement as it meant we also had children on the ward at the same time as adults of all ages. There were pediatric wards in the city, but, because of our designation as the "fever unit," we would still admit children with febrile (fever-related) illnesses of an unknown nature. Almost always, infection turned out to be the cause of illness.

Some months into my house job, I was standing on the ward talking to one of the staff nurses about a patient when a woman, carrying a child bundled in a blanket, burst through the front door and literally handed me the child saying, "She's deathly ill! Please save her." This was not a totally unusual occurrence, as our hospital did not have an emergency room, unlike the other hospitals in the city. This was because most of the referrals and admissions to the hospital came from family physicians who had already seen the patient or been in conversation with the patient or a family member and then made the decision to refer.

It turned out that the mother lived close to the hospital,

and her five-month-old child awoke that morning febrile and, as the mother put it, "not quite right." Over a few hours, the child had become very somnolent, would not feed, and "just went limp." I took the child and, just by looking at her, could see that she was slightly febrile. She felt like a rag doll in my hands. The nurse I had been speaking to ran off without my saying anything, and, in no time at all, a room had been outfitted with a hospital crib for the child. I started my examination even before the bed was ready; clearly, her neck was stiff and she had a fever. As I was examining her, I was speaking out loud. The nurse whom I called for help had already ordered the infant LP kit, being the kind of clinically astute nurse I had become used to in Scotland.

I had now performed quite a few LPs on adults over my months at the hospital, but never on an infant. I mentioned this to the nurse, who nodded her head and came around the examining table on which I was setting things up for the child and the LP.

"I will hold her in my arms and curl her up into a ball so it will be real easy for you. Just remember, you do not have to go very far. She is such a dear, wee thing." I loved the Scotticisms I had become used to over my years in Scotland, and sometimes, but especially at a time like this, hearing them took the pressure off me because there was so much love, caring, and confidence in the sound of the voice and in the words. The child's spine spanned only a half a foot in all, and I could feel the spaces between the bony protuberances very easily. We did the prep quickly; the needle just slipped in with the slight "pop" of the *dura mater*, and out came the turbid-looking fluid.

"Wow! No question what this is—meningitis for sure. We have to find out what kind. Get it over to the lab immediately and have Dr. McGregor call me back with the gram stain." I had already alerted the laboratory doctor, who lived not far from the hospital. He had called the ward to say he had arrived and was waiting for the specimen.

I set up the intravenous and managed to get the needle into the back of the hand. Another technique with which I had lots of practice was putting small needles into small veins, a skill honed when I was a medical student working at the reference laboratory in Copenhagen a few years before. That summer job had me putting needles into tail veins of rats; the rat veins were roughly the same size as the small veins of infants. Soon after the IV was in, there was a call from Dr. McGregor. "H. Influenza—loaded. Come by and have a look." To cover the gram stain findings, I wrote the antibiotic orders for chloramphenicol, a drug with which I was familiar having treated some patients during the tail end of the well-known Aberdeen typhoid fever outbreak the year before. By the time we had everything set up, the mother had returned after having run home to make caregiving arrangements for her other children. She stayed in the room all night. I went over to the lab where Dr. McGregor was cleaning up to go home for the rest of the night. I looked down the microscope at the slide. I could see the bacteria colored red by the gram stain, a short rod-shaped organism teeming with white blood cells around it.

"No question about this, I guess. Even I could make the diagnosis, and I have never seen anything like it since the teaching slides in microbiology."

"We will have the culture results by tomorrow afternoon," replied McGregor. "At least enough to confirm the gram stain, but it's pretty clear what this is."

I dropped in from time to time through the night, as I was on call and awake for most of the time other than short periods when I could lie down but not really get any sleep. Within four hours, the child's color had returned; the fever, which had not been that high to begin with—a common occurrence in severe infections of this kind—was coming down; and her eyes opened for the first time. The night nurse said in her voice of soothing experience to the mother, "She'll be fine. You'll see. She'll be fine. You got her here in time." I got to sleep about four in the morning—eight hours after the child had arrived—and, when I did rounds the next morning at nine o'clock, the child was afebrile (fever-free), awake, and crying with hunger. Sister said, "You've had quite a night. Mom will be back soon to feed her. The child is still at the breast."

The association I had made between the use of chloramphenicol in this childhood case of meningitis and my experience with typhoid fever was partially due to the power of one of my teachers in Dundee. That there were still some chronic typhoid carriers from the outbreak when I arrived in Aberdeen from Dundee soldered the connection. The Aberdeen typhoid outbreak left its mark on the city for at least two years after it ended, because a number of chronic carriers remained, some of whom were receiving treatment at the hospital. I had been exposed to the story of famous typhoid outbreaks in medical school during a lecture on the subject given by our professor of medicine who, after he was knighted by the queen, became Sir Ian Hill. He mesmerized the class with his description of the typhoid outbreak of 1963 at the famous Swiss mountain resort, Zermatt, in which over four hundred skiers from all over Europe were infected. He stood in the front of the class, his small stature overwhelmed by his booming but mellifluous voice, as he slowly and distinctly said "Zermatt." His description of the mountain resort's geography and how the cases worked their way down through the mountain hotels with no apparent initial connection was riveting. The final epidemiological conclusion of waterborne infected sewage seeping into drinking water sources supplying the downstream hotels was a vivid lesson in epidemiological sleuthing that no one in the class would ever forget.

The Aberdeen outbreak that occurred a year later—and

which provided me with my chronic carrier cases from the outbreak—initially had stumped the medical officer of health. Since the cases were spread over the city, the outbreak ultimately became another of the world-famous examples of the careful detective work needed to discover the source of many typhoid fever cases that did not seem to have a focal point as a source. At the time of the outbreak, the various known pieces of information did not seem to add up or make any sense, but eventually all the defined cases were related back to a shop in the center of the city. Aberdeen's then medical officer, Dr. Ian MacQueen, stated: "There is no shadow of doubt that this outbreak started from a tin of corned beef. The meat was in a six-pound can and had come from South America. In an Aberdeen delicatessen it was sliced on a machine that was also used to slice other meats. The infected machine spread the infection to these meats and to the customers who ate them." It was a lesson I learned well: to see and experience in clinical practice what I had only heard of as a medical student, but this time with real patients who could tell me their personal stories. It was a lesson that has never left me.

There was quite a contrast between the acute fever ward and the chest ward at the hospital. In the first, we had all the drama of acute infections of many kinds, as well as strange diseases of which fever was a symptom, but which were not due to infection, such as some malignant diseases and inflammations. On the chest ward, we saw a combination of chronic lung disease and lung cancer. The Scots were big smokers who often acquired the habit when they were ten or eleven years old. You could even buy single cigarettes and "kiddy" packs in some areas to make sure those with limited budgets could get readily hooked. The typical yellow fingers of a smoker were a common finding on teenage hands.

The hack and spit of chronic bronchitis and the pursed-lipped breathing of those with emphysema were a very common observation, not just in the hospital, but on the streets and in the pubs of Scottish towns and villages. Many would talk of smoker's cough as if it were just part of the normal way of life. In the chest ward, we saw the final stages of chronic lung disease with respiratory failure and the most dreaded result of smoking—lung cancer. The ward was a large, old-fashioned Nightingale ward with about thirty beds around a large central area and the nurse's station over at one end. There were curtains that could be pulled around each bed, an improvement over the portable screens that could be set up, but provided less privacy. As the patients who were clearly at the final trajectory of their life became less well and closer to death, we would move them closer to the nursing station so that a sharp eye was available to make sure their needs were met. We used liberal amounts of the Brompton cocktail, which was an elixir meant for use as a pain and cough suppressant. It was named after the Royal Bromptom Hospital in London, England, where the concoction had been created in the 1920s. It consisted of a mixture of morphine, heroin or cocaine, and alcohol, which we, in Aberdeen, supplied as Scotch whiskey. We used it with our terminally-ill cancer patients to relieve pain and the shortness of breath and the coughing fits that plagued them.

One day, the sister called me into her office to speak to the wife of one of our terminal patients. The woman was in tears. "Ian is pining for his dog, Misty, and the dog herself won't eat a thing. She has herded his sheep for ten years, and, since he has been in hospital these past three weeks, it has been awful. I know he is dying, but can he go home for the weekend to say good-bye to Misty?"

It was a fall Thursday, and the cold was beginning to make its way into the buildings, whose heating was not the best. Ian's farm was a two-hour drive from Aberdeen. "Our son can come by tomorrow to pick him up. We will wrap him good and bring him back Sunday afternoon or evening," she said.

I spoke to Sister, "We can do it, can't we? A weekend pass? Can we give him enough Brompton's to get him through?"

"Aye, we can—I have to get permission from the pharmacy to give him a bottle of the Brompton's, but it should be okay. He would be using it here anyway."

"That will be fine, Mrs. McGillivray," she added. "We will have him ready just after lunch and will give you enough medication to get him through the weekend."

On Monday morning when I came to do my rounds, Sister said, "Ian came back yesterday evening, like his wife said he would. He told us he was ready. He spent the weekend with Misty, who would not leave him. But he said his good-byes to the dog and his farm."

When I got to his bed, Ian took my hand and thanked me. "I said good-bye to Misty—I hope she will be okay. My son will take care of her, I know."

Three days later, Ian died, at night, with his wife and son by his bed and the curtain drawn around them. I was not there, but heard from the night nurse that the wife thanked everyone for letting him go to see Misty.

A month later, a parcel in brown paper tied with string and addressed to me lay on Sister's desk. I opened it and inside was a pair of yellow-and-blue Argyle knitted socks with a note from Mrs. McGillivray that said, "We will never forget your kindness to Ian." The socks were a bit rough on the skin the first few times I wore them until they had been repeatedly washed. Whenever I wore them I thought of Ian and his dog Misty. The socks stayed with me for many years as they were virtually indestructible, as had been Ian's spirit.

Chapter 7

The U.S. Army

After I left Dundee and Jeane in 1966, I needed to obtain formal permission from the American government in order to return to Scotland for my house officer's job in Aberdeen. Three days after my arrival back home in Brooklyn, I was in the office of the local selective service board.

"I do not think you can just get another year off. You know there is a war on, and every doctor is needed. You need to serve your country." (Vietnam was raging, and the selective service boards were grabbing every able-bodied male they could find for the draft.) Doctors had a special status, but they were desperately needed as well. This remark was made to me by Mrs. Molloy, the same clerk who had said some nasty things about my studying abroad five years previously when I was applying for my first medical school deferment. Each year she sent me a letter of renewal, and I sensed hostility in every one of them. Now it was full-blown in my face.

"I think you will just have to stay here," she said categorically.

"Is there someone else I can speak to about this? I have this letter telling you that I have been accepted into an internship. Surely you will not stop me from doing it."

"Well, you can just do one over here in your own country. Why should we let you go off to, where is that ... Aberdeen? What kind of place is that? What language do they speak there?"

"Who can I speak to ... in authority ... about this?" I asked.

Her face turned red. She grabbed the phone and dialed, "Colonel Alpert, I have a local fellow who finished his medical studies in ... let me see ... Scotland, who wants to go back for another year. He says he has an internship to do. I told him he must stay here—that whatever he needs to do, he can do it here and then serve his country. He *demanded* to speak to you."

She literally threw the phone receiver at me. "Colonel Alpert, let me explain," I said into the phone. "In Scotland, after medical school ..."

"Do you have an MD degree or not? Just answer me," he bellowed over the phone.

"Colonel Alpert, I have an MB ChB, which in Scotland is ..."

"You are not listening to me. Do you have an MD degree?"

I tried again to explain the nature of my degree and how it was equivalent to an MD degree but not called that, but he interrupted me. "I want you in my office at 9:00 AM tomorrow to straighten this out. Give me back to Mrs. Molloy."

I could hear his voice on the other end as he spoke to her, but not clearly enough to catch the words; she kept nodding in response to orders he was obviously relaying to her. "Here is the address, young man. When you are finished with your interview, please call me so we can make the necessary arrangements for you. I think you will find serving your country to be a very good experience," she said with the faintest smirk on her face.

"I have to be prepared to leave tomorrow, if necessary, and, if I do, I won't be coming back," I said to my parents while checking my passport and packing my bags in preparation for the worst. "I know I could live in Scotland or England. It's a very good place. I can practice medicine there, and you will just have to visit me."

My mother was crying. My father said, "It is a lousy war, and I understand. I wish there was something else we could do. Can you ask him if there is some other service you can do?"

"Dad, he sounded really awful. I don't think I will have a chance to ask him anything. I have to decide on a course of action now so that I am prepared. There is a flight tomorrow night, and my ticket can be changed."

It was a very hot and humid New York summer day. I was at the office building by 8:30 AM, in keeping with my habit of always being early, a habit I attributed later in life to being a premature infant. I would explain to people, "I was two months early at birth, and have never been late since." It always got a laugh, but also established how I looked at scheduling. By 8:45, I was in the colonel's outer office. His secretary pointed to a leather sofa, a bit worn, but quite comfortable. There were American flags everywhere and pictures of men in uniform with various high ranks showing on all the walls. The sign on the door to the inner office read, "Colonel Brian Alpert." This was the office of the Selective Service Bureau - Special Branch and, though I did not know what that meant exactly, it was clearly for people like me. The door was partially open, and I could hear a conversation that sounded friendly, then some laughing followed by some words of farewell. A middle-aged man in a civilian suit walked out, turned, and waved again.

The colonel met me at his door with a paper in his hand. I could see my name on it. He invited me into his office and motioned me to sit down while he went around to his side of the desk and sat in his chair. There was a cigar burning in an ashtray. He looked at me, "Studied in Scotland, it says. I guess you could not get into a good American medical school? But that doesn't matter now. Are you finished?"

I started to explain how medical schools worked in Scotland, figuring I would disregard his question as to why I chose to study there and comment on how good a student I had been at Brooklyn College. I looked up and saw pictures of the colonel in battle dress. I presumed he had been in the Korean War as he did not seem old enough to be a Second World War veteran and still working, but maybe I was wrong. There was a picture of General Eisenhower behind him, signed, "To Brian—Best wishes, Ike."

The colonel looked at me—better yet, glared at me—and said, slowly and distinctly, "Young man, I am not sure if I can call you doctor yet. I want you to answer this question with a yes or no. I do not want any explanations or long-winded discussions. I have a meeting to go to in five minutes and want this settled. Do you have an MD degree—answer me; yes or no—do you?"

I looked at him. Inside brewed an inner imperative to always tell the truth. I had been taught this all my life by the grandmother who had helped to raise me. The colonel had asked me a question to which he wanted an honest and straight answer—either yes or no. "No, sir, I do not have an MD degree." I stopped there, no longer trying to explain the equivalence of the MB ChB degree that I had, or that, in Scotland, an MD degree is a postgraduate medical degree after medical school. "No, sir, I do not."

He looked at me, started getting up, and leaned over the desk, "Well, then, you go back to wherever it is you have to go and get your MD degree, and, when you do, come back and serve your country. Good-bye."

I called Mrs. Molloy and told her what the colonel had

advised me to do. I told her that she would be notified and that I would be coming by for the necessary signature since I was leaving the next day. When I came in the door to her office, she said she had spoken with the colonel. I gave the necessary form for her to sign and left. It was the last time I spoke to her.

A few weeks later, I was on the plane to Glasgow and then on to Aberdeen to start my house job on August 1. During those six months in Aberdeen, I did not think much about the war in Vietnam. Though it was in the British newspapers and on the television news, it was not at the center of my thoughts. I was more interested in learning about infectious disease, rheumatology, and endocrinology—three of the high-volume challenges of our patient population—than in a far-off war. I was also more interested in bedding whomever I could within the limited hours of free time allotted to me as a house officer.

My six months finished without much fanfare, but with enough successes in my medical accomplishments to allow me to feel it had been a good experience. I had learned a lot, performed many medical procedures, and had not done badly socially, though I had failed to convince Lisa, the Norwegian final-year medical student, to take my love for her seriously. I bid her good-bye as I left for Israel to complete my specially organized five-hundred-pound prize internship from Dundee in obstetrics and gynecology at Rambam Hospital in Haifa, where I had been a medical student in 1965.

I was welcomed warmly back into the department and felt as if I were returning to family. Professor Peretz was there, the man who had supervised me during my student visit and who had "adopted" me at that time. The midwives were the same, and they asked me if I would be doing deliveries with them again, to which I nodded yes. The hospital arranged for me to lodge in one of the small bungalows that were set aside for house staff. Esther, the dark-haired, dark-eyed radiography technician with whom I had had a romantic tryst on my first visit, was now on staff and greeted me like a long-lost lover. We had corresponded a bit while I was away, but her command of English was quite rudimentary, making it difficult for meaningful exchanges. But she was exotic looking, and I didn't mind the possibility of having a girlfriend in the hospital.

It was Elana, the *kibbutznik,* with whom I had been most enamored at the end of my previous trip, based a short visit to her kibbutz up north where my Canadian Haifa flatmate's family lived. It had been a three-day visit, and, even though we had shared little physically, I had been taken with her. She fulfilled in me all the romanticized symbolism of the pioneer: strong, beautiful, and single-minded. In fact, she was so single-minded that, after a few letters back to Aberdeen, she asked me if I were coming back to marry her. She told me that, if that was not in my plan, she was being courted by a *kibbutznik* whom she had known all her life, and she would marry him instead. I could not believe that, after so short a visit and without more than a few kisses, she was, in fact, proposing to me. I told her I could not make such a decision but was looking forward to seeing her again when I returned to Israel. A few months later, I received a letter announcing her marriage, with the address of the kibbutz they had moved to in the south. It was on the visit to Elana and her husband at their new kibbutz where, toward the end of my stay in Israel, I met the Indian United Nations soldiers stationed there as peacekeepers who were removed by Abdul Nasser prior to the weeks leading up to the Six-Day War. I traveled to the kibbutz with Yael, the woman with whom I had been staying on my visits to Jerusalem, and whom I eventually married.

I left Israel to visit my sister in Tunisia, leaving Yael with an uncertainty about our relationship and future, and I experienced the Six-Day War through the Arab media. I tried to get through to Israel on my return to London the

day before the war ended, but only managed to finally reach
Yael on the Saturday, the day the Golan fighting ended and
the cease-fire agreement had been signed. East Jerusalem had
been taken by the Israelis four days previously. I was able
to speak to Yael on the phone. It was an emotional phone
call, and she told me they had spent two days in the air raid
shelter but that everything was now okay. I knew I would be
seeing her in New York in a few weeks' time for the marriage
of her sister Daniela to my friend Yoram (the person with
whom I established my first Israeli-Gordon association when I
came as a medical student), his grandparents also being from
Eyshoshuk in Lithuania.

I started my American internship on July 1, 1967, along
with nine other "straights" in medicine (those doing an
internal medicine internship)—all male—plus two senior and
one chief medical resident. Boston University Hospital was
part of the Boston University Medical School with a mixture
of public and private wards, as was common in those days.
The interns and residents literally ran the public wards, and
the attending physicians took on a more or less supervisory
and teaching role. It was quite the opposite on the private
wards, where the attending physicians ran the show and
the interns merely ensured the tests were carried out, and
followed the attending physicians around as they consulted
with their "private" patients. The setup was somewhat alien
to me compared to the egalitarian structure that existed in
Scotland and all the other countries where I had worked
during my years of training, but I was quickly indoctrinated
into the ways of the world of American medicine. The first
time I wanted to order a laboratory test, I was quickly told
that I had to order the complete battery—as that was done by
auto-analyzers and, therefore, much cheaper than single tests.
But, more importantly, as one of my co-interns told me, "It
covers your ass should something go wrong; if you have done
the tests, it is harder to get you into court." I did not quite

grab the concept initially; but, over those first few weeks, I heard the terms "sue" and "court" as the rationale for ordering tests enough times that I began to understand that the threat of lawsuits created an overriding angst among my colleagues.

It was a peculiar summer, getting used to a new system and not being sure about what was going to happen with Yael's visit. I went out with a few of the nurses and a social worker, sure that I could not get into anything serious. No one seemed very interested in a serious relationship anyway.

"Why don't we go to a movie or something?" suggested one of the nurses I had been flirting with, one afternoon. "Are you taken or something?"

I didn't quite know how to answer as Yael was not really a certainty and I did not see anything wrong with going out. "Sure, we can meet after six when I finish doing hand-over rounds." We decided to go out for a meal instead, and she told me a bit about her life growing up in small-town Massachusetts and her admittance into nursing.

"How about coming to my place for coffee?" she asked.

I stammered out a "sure," wondering what I would do if things got heated, as I did not have any condoms; I had not reached the point of even thinking about buying any since my arrival in Boston. I figured, if necessary, we could just neck and play around.

As soon as she closed the door she turned around, grabbed me, and starting kissing me. "You are sweet. I would love to make love to you—okay?" I was dumbfounded. I had never had a woman make such a pass and be so direct with me before. She started taking off her clothes and mine at the same time; she had a studio apartment, so the bed was not far from where we had come in the door. She ran into the bathroom and, a few minutes later, came out naked and jumped into her bed, grabbing my hand on the way. I was feeling very nervous.

"Linda. Look, I don't know what to say, but I don't have anything with me. You know, any contraceptives."

She stopped and looked at me and broke into gales of laughter. "Contraceptives! Have you never heard of the *pill*? *Everyone* is on the pill. Who would use a contraceptive these days?"

"You mean you can be on the pill without being married or having children?" I asked, incredulously.

She looked at me as if I were crazy. "Married? Children? Are you nuts?"

I explained that, when I was in Scotland, the pill was not available by prescription other than for married couples. I may have missed the boat there as I had never pursued it during my last six months, but I did not know any single woman on the pill. She grabbed me and whispered in my ear, "I hate rubbers and I love sex!"

I could not believe it. Only once before in my life had I enjoyed the sensation of unprotected sex—that being with Jeane during our last time together—and that whole encounter had been complicated by all the emotion about virginity and leaving each other, so it had been a bit flat physically, even though very charged emotionally. This was a new experience, and I kept smiling to myself all night and through to the next day after I left for home on my way to work early the next morning. It turned out to be only a two-night stand, but, still, it was quite an experience.

By my second month in Boston, I had heard enough conversations about the various options for military service that I started taking a more active interest in what my co-interns were planning to do the year after our internship finished. I had already received my notification from the draft board and my nemesis, Mrs. Molloy, who I figured was already gloating over the fact that I would be inducted in a year's time according to the normal procedures.

"I think I will enroll in the Berry Plan, do my cardiology, and then do my service. (This plan allowed physicians and surgeons deferment from the draft until they completed their residencies.) Either the war will be over by then, or at least I will be a cardiologist and maybe stationed in a hospital not too near the war zone." That was Ralph, a tall lanky intern from the Midwest.

"I am going to do the same," echoed George, a smooth-talking intern from New Jersey. "I'll do rheumatology. There is a good chance I can stay out of the war zone with that one; not much need for such a specialty in young guys—and it is a nice field—not too many real emergencies."

Morris Alpert, one of the senior residents, gave some advice about choices, and, one day, as a side remark, he added, "I know about this because my uncle is a colonel in the selective service office in New York. He has told me a lot about what you have to do to get the kind of placement you prefer."

Colonel Alpert, I thought. *It must be the same one who had yelled at me to come back with my MD degree.* I did not tell Morris, as I was not sure on which side of the patriot line he stood.

But more and more, I listened and puzzled about the war. I became keenly interested in its progress and started reading everything I could, including *I. F. Stone's Weekly*, sent to me by my father. I was still struggling with the rationale for the Vietnam War when I read Stone's account of what had happened in the Gulf of Tonkin, the event that led to America's entry into the war and which, Stone contended, was mostly fabricated by the U.S. government under President Johnson to rationalize the commitment to the war effort. The more I read, the more I was convinced that this was not a war I wanted any part of, but the issue of what I could do about this remained. Even if I applied for the Berry Plan, should I qualify, it would only give me a deferment and not really satisfy my opposition to the war. I found information about alternatives services such as the National Guard and the Indian Health Service. I applied to the latter in the hope that, if accepted, a couple of years on an Indian reservation would be interesting and would keep me safely away from the conflict. My application was received, and I did a telephone interview with someone who seemed quite interested in my application, so I felt comfortable in this possibility as an alternative to the military.

*   *   *

"My name is Jeffrey Arnold. I am your senior resident. Welcome to the Neurology Department at the Huntingdon Avenue VA."

He was slight in stature, but spoke with enormous authority, weighing his words carefully. I was to be with him for two months—just the two of us and three staff attending physicians. I was given a rapid introduction to the world of VA medicine that first afternoon when I was called to the emergency room for a Second World War veteran with alcoholic brain disease and delirium tremens. I had never seen a case before. I did the workup quickly as the patient had been to the hospital many times before and Jeffrey, as he instructed me to call him, guided me through the treatment of this extremely agitated ex-Marine who was shaking and hallucinating. We used Valium, which was still fairly new, but had replaced the older barbiturate sedatives that had previously been used. I had had very little experience with the drug during my Scottish training years as it was developed while I was in medical school.

"You'll see a lot of alcoholic patients come through neurology—DTs, neuropathies, memory problems. We give everyone who walks into the unit Vitamin B1 just to be on the safe side, even before we know what's wrong with them."

By the second week, I felt more comfortable and had already learned so much from Jeffrey, I could not believe it. The issue of the Vietnam War came up through a newspaper headline, and, when I asked him what he thought, he asked, "What are you going to do?"

"What do you mean?"

"About the draft," he said. "You'll have to do something, you know. I've been through this. I was an Army captain stationed in Washington. I managed to get an honorable discharge as a conscientious objector, but it was not easy to do. What are you going to do?"

This began a long discussion and relationship between us, one that, after receiving word that the Indian Health Service was no longer an option, resulted in my exploring the option of leaving the country rather than responding to my draft obligations, which were to begin July 15, 1968. I had already arranged for the last month of my internship as my vacation, just in case. I knew I could return to the UK, if necessary. I had a provisional license that could be turned into an educational or general license so that I could get more training.

By this time, I was also living with Yael who, after she attended her sister's wedding and we talked, moved in with me in Boston rather than returning to Israel, much to the dismay of her parents. I was not sure exactly what we were doing, but felt moved by the momentum of our deepening relationship, which seemed to follow the terror I experienced during those two days when I believed Israel might be destroyed and Yael along with it. So, we moved in together, renting a basement studio apartment in Kenmore Square in Boston, not far from the famous baseball stadium, Fenway Park.

I took out a book from the hospital library that listed all the medical schools and their teaching hospitals in Canada and noted down the addresses. I wrote to each of them about the possibility of a medical residency in 1968. Then I wrote to my Canadian friend, Chuck, in Montreal—the one with whom I had shared a bungalow in Haifa when I was a medical student. We had kept in touch, and he was finishing dental school at McGill. Yael was not enjoying her time in Boston, and, although my Boston family did its best to "adopt" her, there was not much for her to do as she was not a student, nor could she really find useful work. I was exhausted from work and nights spent on call and not much use when I got home, often falling asleep early on after dinner. So tired was I, that I did not even have much of a desire for sex—she was on the pill, which I had not realized was already commonly used in Israel—but that did not matter much for I had little energy to explore the issue. Between her parents expressing dismay in letters about her staying and interrupting her studies and my own concerns about Vietnam while trying to be an intern with alternate night on-calls, it was not an easy time for either of us. Nor was it, as I found out from some of my colleagues who were willing to discuss their personal lives, for many of the other young couples who were part of the internship program.

The first acceptance letter arrived from the Royal Alexandra Hospital in Edmonton. The brochure describing the hospital and the program was impressive. I took out the map of Canada—having only been to Montreal for Expo 67—and looked for Edmonton. There it was, right in the middle of Alberta, almost in the center of Canada. I looked in an almanac; it was a very cold place! Yael was already having problems with the Boston fall weather, and winter had not even started yet, so I wrote them a letter of thanks, advising them that I would consider the offer and get back to them. According to the offer, I had two months to confirm my acceptance. Two weeks later, an offer came from the Royal Victoria Hospital in Montreal, a McGill University Hospital. It was only a few hours north of New York, or so it seemed on the map. I consulted with Jeffrey, who advised me to take it. The process of arranging to leave the country without anyone knowing of our plans became the next order of business. I understood that making the move would be the end of my status as an American.

"I have to do it," I explained to my parents when they visited. "I can't go to that war, and postponing doing my military service over and over again just does not make sense to me."

My mother was very upset, but added, as if trying to convince herself, "Montreal is not that far away."

"I will not be able to come home if anything happens," I reminded them, "but you will be able to visit me." Yael did not say much. We had not figured out what we were going to do about our relationship, but it looked as if we were gradually drifting into the path of getting married, though part of the decision seemed to come from a concerted feeling of defiance toward her parents … along with a sense of destiny.

*   *   *

It was a cold and snowy January, and, on our wedding day, the car was covered in snow. I called my Aunt Polly, at whose house our wedding was to take place. My parents had arrived two days earlier to help with the arrangements, and were staying there, so at least they would be at the wedding. "I am not sure I can get out of the snowbank," I told her.

"It will be a bountiful life that you will have as evidenced by this show of plenty from heaven." That was Polly, always with a positive view of the world. I managed to get the old Volkswagen out of the snowbank, and we drove through what seemed like a blizzard to Polly's spacious home. Yoram and Daniela had fortunately come the day before from New York so they could attend, as did some close members of my family. Yael's mother and father did not attend, pleading expense and distance as the excuse. Yael wore a nice cocktail dress and used Daniela's veil from her recent wedding in New York. Following the ceremony, we had a social gathering with food at Polly's, and then everyone went separate ways. We went home to our basement studio—married.

Then came the case that served as the wake-up call to me. I now knew I had to leave. Army doctor Capt. Howard Levy was court-martialed for refusing to provide medical training for Special Forces soldiers headed for the war zone. Captain Levy, a thirty-year-old dermatologist from Brooklyn, was convicted of disobedience and seeking to promote disloyalty. He served twenty-six months in prison for the offense. The case resonated with me and others like me. I knew I had to leave the country, and went over my plans with Jeffrey, who had become my confidant and advisor even though I had finished my rotation at the VA. We never spoke on the phone, as I had become very paranoid. In order for me to complete this plan for freedom, I had to apply to Canada for landed immigrant status since merely going there for a residency would not solve the problem permanently. I needed a way of staying in another country legally once my residency was finished. I filled out all the application forms, but was afraid to send them directly to the immigration office in Montreal. Chuck, my Canadian friend, agreed that, if I sent the material to his home, he would hand deliver the papers for me. He also told me that, if it were possible, he would pick up papers from the immigration office and send them to me. This was not always acceptable to the Canadian authorities. Every time an official document arrived from Canada, I trembled, waiting for some FBI agent to barge through the door, even though I knew that, so far, my activities actually did not involve the breaking of any law.

Everything was falling into place. I had received assurances that all efforts would be made to finalize my application in time for me to start my residency in Montreal. Chuck's family offered to put us up until we found a place to stay. By taking my last month of internship as vacation, even though we could not actually leave Boston until the latter part of the month, should anyone stop us along the way, I would be leaving the country within a time frame that I was legally allowed to do so. The anti-war movement was building steam, and reactions by police were often quite violent. I had been told a telegram would arrive. I called the immigration office; it was closed because of a Quebec holiday. We had already packed everything so that it could fit into the Volkswagen. We were ready to leave at the drop of a hat. My parents phoned repeatedly, asking what was happening. It was nerve-racking. I would look out our basement window wondering if we were being watched by the FBI. The phone rang …

"A telegram is waiting for you at the post office in Cambridge." I leaped into the car and almost missed the turnoff to Cambridge. My hands were shaking as I signed for the telegram, daring to open it only once I was back in the car. "This is to provide you permission to enter … landed immigrant from date …" I returned home; we went to sleep and woke at five in the morning. We quickly loaded the car and began our drive north. At the border, in my anxiety, I accidentally almost entered the exit road to the American immigration side, but reversed quickly and went up the other side where the Canadian officials were waiting. I handed them the telegram and our two passports and said, with echoes of what my grandparents must have felt so many years ago when they said the same phrase, "I am seeking entry as an immigrant."

*   *   *

It was July 15, the day I should have been inducted into the army at Fort Hamilton in Brooklyn, a place I had passed many times when driving into Manhattan. I was sitting next to Brian Naibaum, another medical resident from the States (but not a "draft dodger" as people were beginning to call people like me). We were sitting in the dark, listening to grand rounds at the Royal Victoria Hospital, a huge edifice that I was just beginning to get to know well. (Grand rounds are large meetings in which members of the medical staff and medical trainees discuss difficult and challenging cases and new concepts in medical practice.) With some help, Yael and I had found an apartment just a bus ride from the hospital in a nice residential neighborhood not far from one of the Jewish areas in the city. We could walk to a bagel bakery! "Brian, do you realize," I said in a whisper, as the speaker was droning on about some rare disease, referring to the slides on the screen, "at Fort Hamilton in Brooklyn someone is calling my name and I am not there!"

"I know, and you are under arrest!" he said playfully, as he slammed down a pen that happened to be stamped "U.S. Government," a souvenir from his last rotation at a VA hospital. I burst out laughing and was so disruptive that I finally had to leave the auditorium. I was safe in Canada—or at least I felt safe.

A few weeks later, I opened the door to a knock just after dinnertime and found two huge men standing there. One of them showed me an RCMP (Royal Canadian Mounted Police) badge. I was in a T-shirt and jeans. My lips turned dry as I asked them in. Yael was in the living room—our apartment had a bedroom and a living room—a luxury compared to the studio we'd had in Boston. One of the officers said, "Your immigration papers and passports, please. Where are you working, and can you prove it?"

I handed over all the papers and my nametag from "the Vic," as we called it. I also showed them my white jacket with the name of the Vic embroidered on it. "Is everything okay?" I asked timorously as one of them filled out some pages in a book he was carrying.

"Yes, no problem. We have to do this—you know the States. You are in good company; we've done a few hundred of these already. Good night!"

I had already been thinking about how quickly we could escape if we had to, and where we might go. That evening began a process that eventually led us to make plans to go to Israel rather than continue in Montreal for a few more years of training. The French culture was alien to us. The weather proved to be bitterly cold and dangerous for walking, especially for Yael, who could not adjust to the snow, the cold, and the ice. As we started communicating with her parents, who begged us to return home, the idea of immigrating to Israel began to be attractive to me. And then, fortuitously, I was offered a position in Pathology at Hadassah Hospital. The position made tremendous sense, as I knew virtually no Hebrew other than what I had gleaned during my stays in Israel, on top of what I had learned as a child in Hebrew School.

We had time; we had some freedom. My parents were stunned by our decision to leave again, but accepted our decision, just as they had always accepted everything I had done. They had no objections to Israel, but my mother was worried that it was dangerous and very far away.

"You'll see; you'll visit us," Yael assured them. She tried to be welcoming and warm when they visited us in Montreal—she recognized that this was a big move for us, and for them—but for the first time since she had come to North America, I saw her smiling more often, especially as we started the process of deciding what we would take back to Israel.

My parents arranged for us to pick up a Saab with left-hand drive in London. The car was to be a gift from my parents and supposedly, from the write-ups, one that would last us a long time. We meandered around Europe for three months as if on the honeymoon we had never had, staying in student and youth hostels or small hotels, coming to know each other more deeply as we enjoyed each other's company. As we drove around Greece, Yael positively blossomed as she began to recognize the familiar smells and skies of the Mediterranean. We took the boat from Piraeus to Haifa. From the deck, Yael could pick out her parents waving from the dock, and, when we disembarked, there were hugs and kisses all around. Martin, her famous political science father, of German Jewish background and a very formal man, actually embraced me too.

Chapter 8
The Israeli Defense Forces (IDF)

I had forgotten that so many young Israelis were in uniform and carried guns. As we drove through Jerusalem, I was taken aback at the numbers. We were taken to Kiriyat HaYovel, an old neighborhood where Beit Giora, our absorption center, was situated. It was a hot September day in 1969 as we carried our belongings up to the second floor and said good-bye to everyone. The room in Beit Giora was quite small—two single beds, one on each side of the room, a small table, a hot plate, and toilet with shower—with little room for personal items. We were to be there until our apartment, located in an area bordering on East Jerusalem that had previously been a no-man's-land, was ready. We were driven by it the next day. It seemed to be in a desolate part of town outside the main part of Jerusalem, and looked very much like a building site, with only a few finished four-story, walk-up, eight-unit apartment buildings and no trees or shrubbery. "I can't believe this will be ready in three months!"—which is what we had been told—"I guess we will be in Beit Giora for awhile," I said to Yael.

The next morning, I waited at the stop for the bus that went to Hadassah. The bus arrived and, as I stepped in, I could hear a news broadcast on the radio. I could not understand much of it, just a word here and there like *Kol Yisroel*—the Voice of Israel—which was the broadcasting station. At the hospital, I was introduced to the members of the pathology department with whom I would be working: first, Professor Unger, the German Jewish head of the department who, because of a connection from the "old days" with my mother-in-law, had secured me the position in the department as a junior resident in pathology. Michael Goldberg, from Toronto, was a fellow who had completed part of his surgical training at the Mt. Sinai Hospital, and so we bonded immediately because of our Canadian connection. Aaron Polliack, a South African junior staff person, was to be my supervisor, and we clicked right away as well. The rest of the department was a mixture of South Africans and Israelis. English flowed liberally in the department, so much so that I hardly had a chance to use the few words of Hebrew I tried to interject from time to time (which most of the time drew a good laugh). Because of my language limitations, my pathological reports were drawn up in English, and, once approved by Aaron, translated into Hebrew by Esther, the bilingual secretary. Esther ran the department in terms of its ebb and flow and work assignments, determining who would be assigned to surgical frozen sections, regular reporting, or who would perform postmortems. I was given a ten-minute tour of the morgue and introduced to Aslan, who ran the morgue and assisted at "posts" as postmortems were called. "You can count on Aslan. He knows everything. Just listen to him," Aaron instructed me.

*   *   *

The pounding on the door was intense. "Telephone call.

It is Hadassah." The words came first in Hebrew and then in somewhat broken English.

Hadassah at three in the morning; what could that be? I wondered. It was Thursday night. "Yes," I said, when I got on the phone. "Please speak English; I do not understand Hebrew." I said in both English and Hebrew. It was a phrase I had learned quickly in my dealings at the hospital.

"This is the surgical resident. We have an emergency—an unexplained death, and my chief wants a post but we need to do it now—it is an emergency," he repeated again.

I listened and asked, "How can a postmortem be an emergency? I understand surgery being an emergency, but a postmortem? Now that I do not understand." There was a moment of silence.

"You don't understand. It is three in the morning. We have to get the post done before the family arrives on the ward. They won't agree, so, even though we have the signatures of the department head and administrator to go ahead, we will have to do it before the family arrives. Otherwise ... well, you know!"

"No, I don't know. Why do we have to do it before the family arrives—don't you have to obtain their permission?"

"Not if we have the two signatures. I really can't explain—I have to get to the emergency room for an urgent case—please, just come quickly. I was told to tell you that Aslan has already been informed and will wait for you at the entrance to the morgue."

"I have never heard of an emergency postmortem," I said to Yael when I returned to the room to get dressed.

"This is a crazy country, you know," she said in a half-awake voice that had a touch of affectionate humor in it.

A taxi sent by the hospital was waiting for me outside the front door. "To the morgue entrance of Hadassah," I said, in broken Hebrew. Yael had told me the words to say, but the driver already seemed to know exactly where we were going.

"You are going to the morgue? Always early in the morning; always I pick up the young doctors." His English, though broken, was good enough for me to understand that he had done this many times before. "I am from Abu Gosh, not far from Jerusalem," he said. "I do a lot of driving for the hospitals in the city. Me, mostly Hadassah, but also for Shaare Zedek— you know, the old one on Jaffa Road?"

"I don't really know it, but have heard of it. I have just arrived here so do not know my way around very well."

I could see his face in the rearview mirror looking at me. "You will be fine. Jerusalem is a beautiful city. Full of history."

We pulled up to a door at the back of the hospital, out of the way of the main gate. A man with white hair opened the steel door after I rang the bell and spoke through an intercom, saying, "I am Aslan, come in."

It was my first time in a morgue since medical school when we would do pathology rounds with Professor Lendrum. He would test the diagnostic presumptions of the medical registrar as he either confirmed or provided alternative findings to explain symptoms. That had been a real eye-opener for me as to the limits of medical diagnosis, and had laid firmly in my mind the importance of the postmortem, even with the growing sophistication of medical technologies. The morgue smelled of formaldehyde. On the stainless steel table lay the body of a bearded older man.

"Religious. We have to be fast or the family will be upset," said Aslan. "Professor Lastman said he would be here at 6:00 AM. We have less than an hour and a half to get everything laid out the way he wants so he can take the specimens, close up the body, and have it ready for the *Hevra Kadisha*." I looked at him with a questioning eye.

"The burial people," he explained. "They take the body away. I will instruct you, but you must do the cutting. I can but show you where and what. I will take pictures for slides as we open things up." He started reading from a sheet of paper. "It says that the person died five days after successful colon surgery for resection of a cancer. There were no major findings on examination, but there was a high white blood count and they assumed it was a urinary tract infection from the catheter."

The chart was on the table next to the dissecting table, but I could not read the notes. I found the temperature chart and saw the temperatures were swinging up and down. I wondered why they had assumed a urinary tract infection. I could see where antibiotics were started two days before the death with no effect on the temperature. But the rest of the chart was a mystery to me, as the Hebrew words meant nothing, given my complete ignorance of the handwritten language. I had problems enough with the printed language.

I cut down the center of the body as Aslan instructed, and the odor was quite noticeable. There was exuded thick yellowish liquid over the bowel on the left-hand side. I started first with the thorax to be sure I wasn't missing anything. As I moved organs aside, Aslan snapped photos. I wrote down what I could see, but knew that my observations would have to be verified by Professor Lastman. I finished the thorax and thought the heart and lungs looked pretty good, but the bottom of the lungs seemed a bit dense. As I got to the abdomen and started moving the organs around, I could see the anastomosis, the point at which the two parts of the colon had been connected to each other after the cancer had been resected. Surrounding it was a pocket of foul-smelling pus—with some sticky material around it. One of the sutures meant to be holding the two parts together was hanging open. Aslan took some pictures as I moved the organs this way and that so he could get a good angle.

"I think that explains it, Aslan. The anastomosis leaked and there is a pocket of pus—an abscess—which is why the fever did not come down with the antibiotics."

He seemed intrigued. "I think I have seen this before,

but we'd better wait for Professor Lastman to make sure you are right." We looked at the liver and the kidneys in the meanwhile, and then the intercom rang. Aslan confirmed it was the professor and opened the door to let him in.

Professor Lastman introduced himself. His face was round like a cherub's, and he was almost completely bald. We did not shake hands as mine were in latex gloves and covered with bits of tissue. "So what do you have, young man?" he asked in perfect English with a slightly Germanic accent, one I recognized from my father-in-law's manner of speaking and from my travels through Germany as a student. I showed him the surgical site and the abscess.

"Let us take some sections for pathology slides. Aslan, you have the pictures done?" He made a few cuts at the anastomosis and then several of the abscess and surrounding tissues. "Here it is about to erode into the bladder, but he died before it happened. That would have killed him as well. I am taking some small samples from his liver … here you see … I think that is an abscess forming. He probably had septicemia as his final illness. Close up fast before there is any response from the family. It is a good thing we did this, as it means there will have to be a clinical pathological conference. The surgeons never like to hear about these outcomes, but it is important that we do them and inform them of bad outcomes—even when, for religious reasons, the family would prefer that it not be done."

At this point there was banging on the outside steel door. "Let us in; you have taken the body without our permission." Or at least that is what Lastman told me was being screamed at us. "Someone tipped off the family," he said. "It happens all the time. Good thing we got this done in time. Call security, Aslan, and let us close everything up so they can have the body. Assure them that all the body organs are there." A few minutes later, after some quick and large stitches, the body was closed and Aslan took it off the dissecting table. A security guard came to another door and escorted us out of the morgue. We could hear the shouts at the first door, and Aslan yelling something to them through the door.

"You have the samples, Michael? We have to bring them to the department and then we can go. The guard will go with you to the front of the building to wait for the taxi, just in case—usually there is no problem once they hear that the body is ready to be picked up—but it can really be a problem when someone tips them off. Sometimes they come before we can get the post done, and then we just stop. It is too stressful to try and do it with banging and screaming outside the door, and it is just too much hassle to call security. Besides, someone always calls the papers and then it is in the news again, so we try to avoid such scenes. The law allows us to do this with the proper authorization, which we always get, but it is just bad publicity and not worth the bother."

*   *   *

The months went by. There was a terrorist attack in my neighborhood at the bus stop where I daily boarded the bus to Hadassah. Perhaps just fifteen minutes after I caught the bus—running because I was late—a small explosive device went off in a garbage can and severely injured a waiting passenger. We were always being reminded about potential dangers, which caused a degree of anxiety, but there was little one could do. Once, while I was in the Hadassah cafeteria, I noticed a plastic bag left on a chair at an empty table near where I was sitting. I looked around and, when I saw that the table was empty, called the security guard. Within moments, as the cafeteria was being emptied, an older woman came out of a door, running toward the table, saying in Yiddish, "I forgot my knitting bag!" There was a pause as the security guards looked at her and she made a beeline for the table where, on closer examination, I could now see a knitting needle peeping through the top of the bag. There was some tittering from the patrons, who went back to their tables as one of the guards started talking to the woman, likely admonishing her that what she did was not right. She seemed to be more interested in the fact that she forgot her knitting than in the fact that it might have been blown up by the security forces.

*　　*　　*

Toward the middle of December, when the temperature in Jerusalem was getting cold, I received a phone call at the hospital. It was from General Eldar, the Director of the Army Medical Corps. The secretary of the commanding officer told me he wanted to speak to me. We met a few days later.

"How do you like your pathology training?"

"It's okay—it works for me now because my Hebrew is not great—my passion is internal medicine, and I will return to it after I get settled. We are still living in an absorption center. My wife is back at university."

"How would you like to do your military service a bit earlier than you have to? I know that you can wait at least a year, maybe even two, depending on where you are in your residency training. But, if you agree to join up in one month in January, I can guarantee you a medical posting on an air base. We are looking for a few doctors with a bit more experience than those who usually go into the service right out of an Israeli internship. I see you have done two internships and a year of medical residency. You may not know this, but a stationing on air base is the best of all positions. You will have a house so your wife can stay with you, and there is always a swimming pool on the base, a supermarket, and an officers' club. You could probably visit your home every other weekend. It is really very nice."

"And if I choose to wait?" I asked.

"No problem; there are armor, artillery, and infantry bases

all through the Sinai that would love to have you. And you could get back into the country proper every few weeks with a bit of luck—your choice, of course."

"I have to talk it over with my wife. May I have a few days to think about it?"

"Sure. Call me next week."

It was a quick decision after Yael gave me the lowdown on military service and what it meant to be in the air force. But mostly it was because I was quickly becoming bored with pathology and could not see it leading anywhere. Added to this, no matter how hard I tried, I was not learning any Hebrew because everyone in the department spoke to me in English.

I called Eldar back and said, "I have decided yes. What should I do?"

"Your papers will arrive next week, with the base you will report to and the time and date listed on them. Good luck— you've made a good choice."

I said good-bye at the department. They even had a little good-bye party with lots of good wishes and toasts to my health and a successful service. Two weeks later I arrived at Bad Arba (Base Four in Hebrew), halfway between Jerusalem and Tel Aviv. I was issued my uniform, and we gathered in a large classroom—we being a mix of immigrant doctors like me from all over the world, and a number of Israelis who chose to do their military service after medical school rather than before. Although everyone spoke some English, the language of instruction was Hebrew. Within the first few days, I had connected with two doctors—one an Argentinean and one an Israeli—as buddies. Because of how our names fell after each other alphabetically, we were often in the same groups for activities.

The lectures were a challenge—I could hardly understand them—but wrote down as much as I could phonetically and, later at night, with Yael's help, would figure out the substance of the lecture. Some of the practical courses were easier as I had considerable experience in emergency medicine. Even with my limited Hebrew, I could usually handle anything to do with acute emergency care, as much of the talk was in universal "medicalese." I excelled at setting up intravenous infusions, putting in catheters, and dealing with fractures and bleeding. I also held my own in the military practical tasks. Because of my background in engineering from Brooklyn Technical High School and growing up in a household with an engineer father, I had always loved to take things apart and put them back together again. This made it relatively easy for me to win the prize for the speed in which I disassembled and reassembled my M16 rifle, including an exercise when we performed the task with our eyes blindfolded. The Uzi was a quick learn, as was the Beretta pistol I was issued for the course. In spite of the language disadvantage, although I knew I wasn't grasping everything, it was comforting to know that I was no worse than some of the other foreign-born doctors.

We were loaded into a large truck early one morning, having had to report to the base by 5:00 AM. We slept home at nights—there was no provision for the doctors to sleep at the base—and those who lived far away would stay with friends or family close to the base. Luckily, I had a car so I could drive in from Jerusalem in the morning, but this day the call to duty was very early.

"We are going into Nablus for an exercise. There have been some problems there from time to time, but we should be okay. After we get through the town and arrive at our destination, you will be given instructions. You will be expected to read the terrain maps and get from where we drop you off to the gathering spot. You will be fully armed and carrying the equivalent of a full combat medical pack—about twenty-five kilograms."

This was from the commander, who was an Argentinean doctor, a hero who had lost his arm in a battle with terrorists at the Jordan border a couple of years before while helping to extract some of the wounded soldiers in his unit. He was now a course instructor, and he spoke Hebrew with a heavy Spanish accent. When it was clear from the look on my face that I did not understand something, he would translate into English, but that was equally imbued with a thick Spanish accent. I sat at the back of the truck and was given a semi-automatic modification of the M16, with two clips of bullets. On the ride there, Ariel (his adopted Hebrew name)—my Argentinean buddy—was next to me. He, too, had been issued the same rifle. Half the guys were asleep, but Ariel and I kept looking back to where we had come from, so we knew when we had entered the West Bank.

We were following a jeep in which the commander was riding. We stopped at the entrance to Nablus when the commander came around to the back of the truck and woke everyone up. "Get ready! We are entering the town. Be prepared for anything. Sometimes they try to sabotage these exercises and throw hand grenades at the vehicles."

I was listening carefully and caught most of what he was saying. He looked at the two of us sitting at the back of the truck and told us to take our guns off safety and make sure we had the second clip handy. He then said something rapidly, which I was slowly translating to myself when he jumped off the bumper on which he had been standing. "If anyone moves suddenly behind the truck, enter into him a ball! (He had used a word for ball that I did not realize was also used in slang to mean bullet.)

I turned to Ariel and said, "Enter into him a ball?"

He looked at me with a big smile and said, "Shoot. Anyone moves, shoot him!"

A shudder ran down my spine. Shoot him? I knew how to use the gun and, on semiautomatic, I could shoot a lot of bullets pretty quickly—a squeeze each time for a burst of three bullets—but I had never thought about shooting a person.

What did "anyone moves behind the truck" really mean? What if someone decided to throw a stone? Was that a reason to shoot? I checked the safety again; it was off, and twenty bullets were in the magazine. I was very nervous and, I can admit now, maybe even a little scared.

We passed through the town without incident. I put the safety back on my gun. We unloaded our gear, got our maps out, and broke into groups of six. Three hours later, after traversing some steep hills, we arrived, an hour ahead of schedule. We set up our field treatment unit as directed and broke out the K-rations. To my delight, among other highly caloric foods, our lunch contained *halvah*, a sweet made from ground sesame seeds and honey. It had been one of my favorite treats long before I came to Israel. Everyone agreed that the *halvah* made the whole exercise worthwhile as we each packed it away.

Three weeks later, I received my *darga* (rank)—two cloth stripes to put on my uniform. The single bar of a second lieutenant would be given to me only when I arrived on the air base and received my air force uniform. I drove into the base, Hatzor—also known as *Kanaf Arba* (Wing Four)—en route to Beersheva and reported to the base commander. He spoke to me in English after I told him my Hebrew was not great. I gave him my short history as we talked. "I don't really care all that much how good your Hebrew might be; what I care about is how good a doctor you are. Are you a good doctor?" He was a general—though at this time I wasn't quite sure how high up the ranks he was—but more importantly, he was my base commander. I looked at him and replied, with some inward trepidation, "Yes, I am. I have only had a few years of training, but have been considered good wherever I have trained. I *am* good, but know that I can always be better, and will always try to be good and better." He looked at me and stood, shook my hand, and said, "Welcome to Hatzor."

For the first few months, there was no house, even though Dr. Eldar had promised I would have one. I had a small room to myself, but no place where Yael could stay comfortably. But, within a few weeks of starting my service, our apartment in Jerusalem was finally ready, and we took possession. It was quite lovely, with a view that overlooked green hills and valleys. We had west-facing windows, and every night there was a glorious sunset of the kind that one sees often in Israel, unexcelled anywhere in the world. Young trees had been planted in the neighborhood, and, although the area still looked like a building site in some parts, it was beginning to take shape. Our neighbors in the building were mostly young families: a combination of Moroccan, Argentinean, and South African. It was easy to be neighborly with the mix, and, when I started coming home in uniform, I was always greeted very warmly.

"Your house is ready," the base operations officer said to me one day as I passed him coming out of the dining room. "You can move in after Shabbat." By this time I was able to converse reasonably well in Hebrew, though with a limited vocabulary. I was learning it in the clinic which, as the base's junior doctor, I ran every morning. The senior doctor held two afternoon clinics, attended to other administrative duties, and—as I soon learned—also moonlighted off the base three afternoons a week. At the first clinic I attended, I was introduced to the *hovshim* (the plural of *hovesh*—medic) who would be my right and left hands in all things related to running the base's medical service. Ovid was the chief *hovesh*, a Yemenite with a smile that would brighten any room. We agreed that he would speak to me only in Hebrew unless it was an emergency and there was something I didn't understand. In this fashion, day to day, I would learn Hebrew in the clinic—the *hovshim* did not speak English or, as in this agreement, refused to speak it other than when requested by me to do so because I was in a jam.

My main assistant hardly spoke English at all, and she vowed to teach me Hebrew by acting out words. As a result, to an outsider, our work together often appeared as a game of charades. As a new word came up, I would write it down—phonetically first; and then with Hebrew letters—under the tutelage of Nahama (my only *hoveshet*, which is a female *hovesh*), who sat by my desk during the clinic interviews. The first prescription I wrote was for a skin cream, which she explained to me by vigorously rubbing her arms up and down while saying "*mishcha, mishcha*" (ointment or skin cream). It worked. First my medical vocabulary grew, and then my regular vocabulary grew day by day.

*　　*　　*

In addition to the enlisted soldiers, I also looked after the officers, the pilots, senior officers, and their families—mostly wives and children—as only a few of the more senior officers were married women. In an effort to ingratiate myself with the children, I bought a supply of lollipops and, after each house call in which I examined a child, I would give the child a lollipop. According to my expanding Hebrew vocabulary, I thought the word for lollipop was *sukkerit al makel*, with *makel* being a stick, and *sukkerit* a candy, or so I believed, coming from the root letters for sweet. I had learned that Hebrew words were all built from three-letter roots, and that one could learn and build words based on those three letters (with *skr* being the three for sugar and, therefore, according to my logic, all things sweet).

My ploy seemed to work, and, as I gave out the lollipops saying in Hebrew, "Here is your *sukkerit al makel*," I would always get a smile from the child and, often, a good laugh from the mother, which I took as a positive affirmation of my mastering Hebrew. One day while visiting the home of the wife of one of the base's star pilots, Eitan Ben-Eliyahu, after giving her child a lollipop and receiving the accustomed, positive smile and laugh, she said in Hebrew, "Dr. Michael (as

I began to be affectionately called), we all like you very much and think you are a very nice person and a good doctor. That is why I have been asked by the mothers to tell you that, even though we have been enjoying it very much, you have been using the incorrect word for lollipop. The word for lollipop is *succharia al makel*. What, in fact, you have been saying is "diabetes on a stick" since the word *sukkerit* is the sugar illness—you know ... diabetes." She gave a big smile and I had to laugh—not just because of my understandable mistake, but because all the wives had been keeping it from me because it was a good collective laugh. I thanked her, looked at her child, took out another lollipop, and said in my best Hebrew, "Here is another *succharia al makel*." She gave a big clap and wished me a good afternoon as she closed the door behind me.

*   *   *

As time passed, I got into the swing of things at the base, finally being introduced into the moonlighting system, which gave me the use of a car and gas coupons from the local health authority. When I moonlighted, I covered the local *kibbutzim* (agricultural communes) and *moshavim* (farm cooperatives). It was interesting and varied primary care as each community had its own special ethno-cultural mix—North African, Yemenite, South African, Latin American, and American—each with a history and culture. At each location, I worked through the local nurse, who usually lived in the community and acted as the primary care person. Without her, it would have been impossible to function: many of the communities were quite rural, and the closest town could be as much as an hour away from a rural community where there may not even have been many cars for transportation. By public transportation, the trip could take two or more hours. One of the *moshavim* was right outside the air base; this one was the easiest to service. Also, one of the most adept nurses lived there.

"Quick, go out to the runways," Ovid said. "They are coming: the F4s, the Phantoms!" This was a few weeks after I had started working on the base and had started feeling part of the family. As yet, I had not been to the hangers or runways to see the base's planes up close. I knew we had Sky Hawks and Phantoms—with the latter being a bit of a secret—or so I thought. Another group of four F4s was being delivered to the base; the first planes had landed on September 5, a few months previously, while I was still working in Jerusalem. (During my employment at Hadassah, I had noticed that each paycheck had a tax withheld—the so-called "Phantom tax"—to pay for airplanes, something I did not understand completely except that it resulted in my *netto* being lower than my *brutto* (the amount at the top of my paycheck before all the deductions were taken off).

I ran across the path that led from the living areas where the duplex bungalows (of which ours was the first in the path) had been built so they were closest to the clinic, and then down to the hangers, but not to the actual airfield, around which barriers had been set in place. The roar of the planes was enormous: the four planes first flew over the base, some doing fancy maneuvers before coming in to land. Two of them flew in very low and then peeled back and shot straight up instead of landing. More would arrive over the next few months until the base had its full squadron. I was taken by my neighbor—the wing commander—to see them up close. They were huge, with room for a pilot and copilot, and they dwarfed the other planes on the base.

The routine on the base was well established: morning clinics and afternoon house calls. These visits always resulted in some kibitzing with the wives of the pilots. I also had a few afternoons moonlighting once I was brought into the program by the Regional Health Authority. The use of the car—not to mention the extra money—was most welcome as my officer's pay was not very much and Yael was back at University. We decided to rent out one of the rooms in the apartment in Jerusalem, and that, too, helped defray some of our expenses.

When I was alone on the base during the week, I would often go to the control tower and sit with the crew whose task it was to guide the planes in their nighttime sorties. The War of Attrition was in full swing, and Hatzor was one of the main bases from which attacks were initiated—mainly at the Suez Canal region, but also at the Jordanian border and inland, where their radar bases assisted the Egyptians in their attacks and missile defense systems. I would watch in awe as a nineteen-year-old woman gave orders to seasoned pilots as their F4s took off, the ground shaking and the light blazing as the afterburners roared with enormous heat and light. I would listen to the radio communication, sometimes recognizing one of my neighbors and friends talking about being shot at by anti-aircraft fire or hitting their target and returning to base.

One late afternoon, the news came to my house. My immediate neighbor, Yigal Shochat—the person with whom I shared the duplex and with whom I had spent many evenings along with his wife and child—had been shot down. The news was that he had survived, but, a few days later, we were informed his copilot had died. When Yigal was finally repatriated, in severe kidney failure with a gangrenous leg, we all felt he would likely die. Miraculously, he was saved and, although missing one leg, went on to study medicine, and later became the chief medical officer of the Israel Air Force.

*   *   *

I was sitting in the house of Ran Peker, who had replaced Shmuel Hetz as the F4 squadron commander after Hetz's plane had been tragically shot down. I was having coffee with his wife when Ran came running in, saying, "I cannot tell you what happened, but I cannot believe it! You will hear soon. They cannot fly. They cannot fly!" He was so excited. It was July 30, 1970, some six months after I had started my stint at the air base. That evening, we heard on the news that there had been a direct clash between Israel pilots and Egyptian Air Force planes flown by Russian pilots, which resulted in the downing of five Russian MiG-21s—two at the hands of Israeli Phantoms. What Peker had actually been excited about when he'd come running so excitedly into the house was that the Russian pilots were not much better than their Egyptian counterparts when it came to air-to-air combat. A few days later, just outside my bungalow—on the path leading into the pilot neighborhood—I heard our new base commander, Rafi Harlev, and the commander of the air force, General Mottie Hod, talking about an impending cease-fire. I sat up in bed—it was just under the window—and listened to the conversation, which, though almost at a whisper, I could still hear in the quiet of the early morning. As if in confirmation, on August 7, 1970, Israel and Egypt signed an armistice agreement, bringing an end to the War of Attrition.

*   *   *

It was six in the morning when the phone rang. "Hurry, hurry, there has been a terrible accident on the base. A jeep turned over. Hurry!" It was unusual to receive such calls from the clinic. Even though I could have run there, I drove to the clinic, figuring I might need the car. The *hovesh* on duty was there, another had just woken up, and Ovid was running up the road, his feet flying.

"He turned over his jeep on his last night of watch duty—he was to be discharged today. He is having trouble breathing. We got the suction machine and it is being set up—here it is!" A young sergeant was on the examining table, with terrible face and head injuries. He was struggling for air.

"Cut off his entire shirt so I can see everything," I ordered in a loud and forceful voice.

Ovid was unpacking sterile dressings and had started wiping off the blood covering the soldier's face and mouth. I could hear the sergeant's strident breaths and see that his chest was barely moving as he vainly tried to breathe, with some indrawing of the muscles of his chest, a sign of an airway blockage.

"His airway is obstructed—suction him as much as you can!" I yelled. I regained my composure, knowing that calm worked best in urgent situations. "Ovid," I said as deliberately as I could, "we have to do a tracheotomy. I have never done one. I know there is a special kit. Call for a medivac and explain to them that I am going to try to do the tracheotomy, but they may have to intubate or do a tracheotomy when they arrive and before they take off, so they should have everything ready." (A tracheotomy is a cut through the front of the neck into the trachea or windpipe—the main air passageway in the throat that leads through the bronchi to the lungs. Intubation is the insertion of a breathing tube into the trachea through the mouth. The patient accesses air through the tube.)

"Did you hear what the doctor just said? Call in for a medivac with those instructions," Ovid directed the second *hovesh*, who was next to the phone and the walkie-talkie. He laid out the tracheotomy kit. "Doctor, you will be fine. You know how to do this! I will give you the scalpel and the cannula—the airway is in place already, and the oxygen is ready to go—just relax and do what you know how to do!"

I looked at Ovid, his face full of confidence as he nodded at me to begin. He helped me put on my gloves quickly and swabbed the front of the neck with iodine and alcohol. He pulled the head back for positioning, and I found the thyroid cartilage and felt the tracheal rings below it. Then, I took the packaged scalpel that he held for me so I could pull out the handle with the blade already in place. "Ovid, I am cutting here! If we are lucky, there will not be too much blood as we will be in the midline, but, just in case, have lots of gauze ready to wipe it clean so I can insert the cannula."

The scalpel sliced through the skin, and I could feel the give of the cartilage. There was a small amount of blood, but, more importantly, a rush of air—even with the space not yet opened. I opened the space when I quickly inserted the cannula through the incision, and then twisted it so the hole was of maximum circumference. Immediately, the air rushed in and out, and the young man's chest started moving. I had put the plastic suction tube down the cannula, and blood came up—but the air was moving—I suctioned a few more times until little was coming up. We put the oxygen over the tracheotomy and raised the pressure up to maximum. Now, at least, he could breathe.

I could not see what kind of damage had been done, but he had a severe laceration on his scalp. We had stopped the bleeding with pressure. I was fairly sure there was a depression of the skull at the laceration site. His eyes were closed, and his pupils seemed dilated, but there was no time to examine him. He was not responding to his name when called. I could hear the helicopter coming close—we radioed that the tracheotomy was in place, so they would only have to transfer and lift off. We moved the soldier onto a stretcher and waited just outside the clinic, a few feet from the helipad that had been placed next to the clinic for just such eventualities. Ovid had written up the events and torn off the sheet, leaving the carbon copy for us. The medivac *hovesh* took one of the stretcher handles and another jumped out to take the other side. They deftly lifted the sergeant into the helicopter, and then took off. It was almost as if it had all taken place in one slow-motion picture.

"Ovid, I cannot thank you enough for your help."

"Doctor," he said, "You did it like you had done a hundred before," he said, flashing me his special Ovid smile. The two other *hovshim* patted me on the back, and, as they were cleaning up, started talking about the sergeant whom, of course, they all knew. Ovid called the commanding officer and told him that the sergeant was on his way to the hospital. The family was then called with the news. Later, Ovid would call the hospital every few hours for updates. The sergeant was on a respirator with a very bad head injury. Unfortunately, he died the next day. It was a tragic day for the base and for me—my first major injury. Until that time, any medivacs that I had done each month when I went to the Sinai Peninsula for my on-call medivac service had been simply for illnesses or minor road or work accidents. This was the first soldier I had lost under my command, and it affected me deeply.

*   *   *

Some of my experiences with young, enlisted soldiers were quite humorous. They would do their best to try and get an extra day off if they could, and, before Friday, there would be always be a series of requests for time off due to one fabricated illness or another, the intention being to set up a weekend in Tel Aviv. I recall one young and recently married corporal who tried to explain to me why it was so important for him to have the Friday off because of his bad back. This was one of the more common complaints because soldiers believed it was easy to feign the symptoms—and the required rest was always just a few days—or so they believed. This particular corporal who "limped" into the office, holding his back and grimacing in pain, indicated that he needed time to rest his back and that the Friday off would work well since he would then have Saturday to rest as well. After I took the history, I told him to go into the adjoining examining room and get up on the examining table so that I might examine him.

Without him realizing it, I was then able to observe him "painfully" entering the room and then—when he assumed I could not see him—literally leap onto the table like a gymnast, without any evidence of discomfort. Now able to demonstrate the absence of signs that one might see in a significant back injury, I advised him that I would prescribe some medication and that he could remain on the base since there was no indication for sick leave. He looked at me and the female medic and said, with a slight wink in his eye, "Doctor, I must be home for Friday night. You know, it is Friday"—he looked at me with a knowing expression—"it's a *mitzvah* (a good and holy act) on Friday night," at which point the *hoveshet* blushed and he smiled broadly at me. I realized that he wanted to go home and make love to his wife, with Friday—Shabbat—a special time to do so. I looked at the *hoveshet*, whose blush had settled. She shrugged a bit as I wrote out the permission slip to give him the weekend off for backache and *rest*. When I saw him after the weekend, he gave me one of the biggest smiles I could ever have imagined. Miraculously, his walking was clearly free of pain.

*   *   *

The call came at five in the morning, telling me to come to the clinic. One of the soldiers who had been on guard duty was acting very peculiar; in fact, the *hoveshet* who called termed his behavior "hysterical." It was a brisk walk over to the clinic, where I found a young soldier screaming that there was something in his head that was "making him crazy." On questioning, he admitted that he had fallen asleep in one of the peripheral ditches surrounding the territory he was to guard, and that he had woken up with a terrible feeling in his head. His commanding officer was called, who brought him to the clinic, all the while thinking it a ploy on the part of the soldier to avoid punishment for sleeping during his watch.

Yet, the soldier would suddenly start screaming and hold his hand to his head, always on the left side. Nahama, who was the *hoveshet* on call, said to me in a whisper, "*Yesh lo juk ba rosh,*" which meant, literally, "he has a cockroach in his head"—the colloquialism for "he's crazy." I started the medical examination and, while using the otoscope to look in his ears, noticed the tail end of a black cockroach in his left ear. Every now and then it would wriggle, and, when it did, the soldier screamed for dear life.

"Yes, Nahama," I replied, "you are right: he definitely has a cockroach in his head! Take a look!"

Peering through the otoscope for a look, she let out a cry of amazement. I tried to get the beast out with tweezers, but each time I inserted the instrument in the man's ear, the cockroach would move, the soldier would scream, and all I could get out was a small piece of the wing or foot. "Get me the ethyl chloride spray," I said to Nahama, who brought over the bottle which was used generally to freeze the skin before lancing a boil or pulling out a superficially embedded foreign body. "Just give me a minute. This will feel cold," I said to the soldier, who was in tears. A minute after I administered the spray, I could see that the insect was frozen and now immobilized so that I could catch on to it with the tweezers without it crumbling. I pulled it out, triumphantly holding up the victory prize—one, whole, entire, black inch of it. I showed it to the soldier who threw his arms around me shouting, "*Toda, Toda*" (thanks, thanks) as I turned to Nahama and said, "He really did have a cockroach in his head!"

*   *   *

It was also while in the service that I was finally able to express humor in Hebrew for the first time. Not being able to express myself in a humorous way had been one of my greatest problems. It took me so long to translate what I wanted to say from English into Hebrew as rapidly in my head as I could manage, the ability to say something humorous was invariably lost, either because of insufficient vocabulary or excessive processing time.

We had just picked up General Chaim Bar-Lev, the military commander in chief of the Israeli Defense Forces. We were going to examine the Bar-Lev line, which had been named after him, the first line of defense against the Egyptians at the Suez Canal. The rule was that, when a high-ranking officer needed to be shuttled for such an exercise, a full medivac helicopter and crew, including some support paratroopers, would accompany him. I had previously been on such a flight with Ariel Sharon, who had not spoken to anyone on the helicopter other than the pilot—and much of what he said had to me sounded like instructions, observations, or opinions. From the moment he stepped in, there was a different tone and demeanor with Bar-Lev. He asked all members of the crew their names and where they were from, then sat back and started reading a newspaper that he had with him. After about twenty minutes, he turned around and asked me in Hebrew, "Would you like the paper, doctor?" My head raced as I tried to formulate an answer, reflecting on the fact that I could barely read any Hebrew, much less a newspaper. With rapid internal translation I replied in my best Hebrew, "No, thank you, sir. By the time I would finish reading a newspaper, it would no longer be news ... but history!" He smiled at me and, once he had ascertained how recently I had immigrated to Israel and how quickly I had joined the service, he said, "*Kol Hakavod*" (all due honor and respect) and, instead, handed the paper to one of the medics.

*   *   *

My tour of duty was coming to an end in a few months. The first flight surgeon's course was being organized. Until then, air force physicians had been trained informally and on the job. It was a bit unstructured, especially the medivac and emergency treatment parts of our duties. Looking after pilots was a considerable challenge, but one with which we all had to learn to deal. They were the cream of the crop of the Israeli military, and many had a very high opinion of themselves—some of this high opinion was well deserved in view of their combat experiences and achievements; yet some, perhaps, was not so much deserved. One day, Aaron, one of the most senior pilots—a high-ranking officer—came into the clinic and threw his immunization card on my desk. "Doctor Michael, I need you to sign this so I can go to the U.S. for some special flight training," he said in a playful but somewhat authoritative manner.

I looked at the card and saw that he was missing a smallpox vaccination. "Aaron," I said, "you need your smallpox vaccination. I can do it right here tomorrow. I will have to get the material from the central pharmacy—we do not keep it in stock as there is not much call for it normally. The vaccination itself will only take a couple of minutes."

"Doctor, why don't you just sign it and get it over with? I am sure it is no big deal. Whoever gets smallpox these days?"

"Major ..." I retorted with a warning tone, emphasizing his rank rather than his name, for we were now dealing with serious business, and I did not want to leave this as an exchange between "friends."

"I hate needles," he said, continuing in a more authoritative manner. "I know you are the doctor, but you are also a lieutenant, even if a first lieutenant. As you know—and as you, yourself, said—I, on the other hand, am a major and a veteran pilot. Let's just get this signed."

I had never had anyone pull rank on me before; and I knew that the rules on the base were quite clear: the doctor, regardless of rank, was in charge in all matters related to health. This authority extended all the way up to the base commander, who was a general.

"Major, let me check with the base commander and, if

he says I should follow your request, I will consider it. But I will also have to get the okay from my commander, the chief medical officer of the air force, Colonel Benny Kallner. You know who he is—I believe he delivered both of your children."

He came back the next day, and I administered the smallpox vaccine, which took barely a moment. He hardly felt it, and left with a meek smile on his face, his immunization card signed.

*   *   *

"You can do the course even though you are soon going to finish your service. Since you will be moving on to reserve duty, having the course will be useful for you." This was the message on the phone from Kallner. I was delighted. He followed with, "I know you are American. The only flight surgeon's manual of any use to us is the U.S. flight surgeon's manual. I am not sure how to go about getting it for the course or even if that is at all possible. Would you know anyone you could ask about it?"

I could not believe the synchronicity of the question. He could not have known that my father was a retired engineer who had worked for the Department of Defense and had access to all kinds of reference material and books. In fact, he was a technical writer and had even written some of the manuals that were available through the nonclassified military press. I called home. Because I called so rarely, I immediately told my father that there was no emergency and that everything was okay. I explained what I needed, and, the next day, he called back to tell me that the only thing with the subject matter that Kallner had asked for, and that he could find twenty copies of, was the navy flight surgeon's manual. "It says on the blurb that is the same as the air force one, other than special chapters on aircraft carrier issues."

"Can you order twenty and send them to me at the base—by air mail or as fast as you can send it?" I asked him, delighted that he had found what we needed. Three weeks later—a week before the course was to begin—a large box containing the books arrived. Kallner sent his driver to pick them up. I kept one for myself to start reading before the course began.

Over the course of the training, I sat in the backseat of a trainer flown by Kallner—who was a pilot as well as a doctor—and experienced G-forces, pulled some of my classmates out of the sea from a helicopter hovering overhead, organized mass casualty treatments for an air base, practiced putting intravenous lines into a bouncing helicopter simulator, did medivacs at night, and organized blood transfusions in near total darkness. I learned about high-altitude physiology and problems pilots would face if they bailed out into the sea or were stranded in the desert, how to keep them flying if they were sick, and how to ground them against their will. They agreed to let me do the final examination as an oral since my writing skills had not improved much over the year and a half in the service, despite the best efforts of my *hovshim*. With a touch of irony, I would say my writing was "first grade," but really meaning first grade in school. Kallner had looked at me when I made the request, thumbed his well-worn copy of the naval manual, which I had given to him, and agreed. Two days later he gave me my certificate and shook my hand, saying the traditional, "*Kol Hakavod*"—all honor and respect.

*　　　*　　　*

I had not quite two weeks to go. We were packing up the house and had given notice to the students that we were moving back to our apartment in Jerusalem. I was booked to start my medical residency at Shaare Zedek on July 1, 1971. On May 27, our first child, Neta, had been born in Hadassah

Hospital in Jerusalem. She had spent the first month of her life on the air base, apparently unfazed by the sound of jet fighters, and benefiting from the endless advice that the wives of all the pilots felt it was their duty to provide to Yael.

A week after I returned to the base following the flight surgeon's course, Eitan Ben-Eliyahu came up to me and shook my hand. "Congratulations on completing the course. How would you like to go up with me now that you are a *real* flight surgeon?"

"What do you mean, go up?"

"In an F4—backseat, of course. I have to do a test flight after servicing. You know, take it through its paces, its maneuvers. And for that I do not need the weapons control navigator, so the backseat is open, if you'd like to come."

I could not believe it—this was not flying in a trainer, which I had just done—but in the premier plane of the air force with one of its best pilots. "When?" I asked.

"Day after tomorrow—eight o'clock in the morning. Be there at seven so we can gear you up and explain the G-suit and the eject maneuvers. Don't eat," he warned. "I will give you a bag, but throwing up your breakfast is not a good idea— you have a mask on throughout the flight, and it would mean I'd have to cut things short."

I was so excited I could not sleep that night, but did manage a few hours the night before the flight, only because I knew I had to get some rest. All through my clinic there was nothing else I could think about. Word got around, and everyone was asking me about it. "Where are you going to fly? Do you think you can stomach it? It can go to almost Mach 2, and the G-forces are unbelievable!" None of the comments helped me, but I knew they came from a sense of camaraderie.

"Michael," explained Eitan, "the principles are simple and not all that different from what you learned when flying in the trainer. The G-suit is a lot more complex and will adjust as needed when I accelerate and climb or dive, but you still have to do the muscle and breathing maneuvers you learned in the trainer—remember?"

I had learned and practiced quickly breathing in and out and expelling my breath for several seconds against the closed vocal cords while, at the same time, tightening my leg and stomach muscles as much as I could. It was the Valsalva maneuver, which we had all learned about in medical school and that any woman who has given birth naturally would understand, since it is the push that expels babies. We suited up, and he showed me all the pockets and where things were in case we had to eject. I was helped into the backseat: the tubes were attached to the suit, the helmet put on me, and the oxygen mask adjusted so that, when we were ready, I could affix it easily.

Eitan came over and said, "You see this lever above your head, with the two circles? If you hear me yell "eject," you pull it down with both hands; or if you see me eject, you pull it down and count five seconds. If that does not work, then you pull up on these two handles by the side at the same time. And if that does not result in your ejecting … well, can I have your car?"

He smiled a wide smile and looked over at my blue Saab, which all the pilots loved as it was made by a Swedish company that also made fighter aircraft. He tapped my helmet with his hand and said, "Don't worry; just listen to my instructions, keep your eyes on the instrument panel, and hang on."

The roar and rumbling sound from within the plane was like nothing I was used to hearing from the outside. It grabbed my whole body. I looked to the left as we streaked past the control tower. I had seen scores of F4s take off, their afterburners blazing blue and yellow flames and black smoke. As we lifted off, I could feel the slight tug of the G-suit around my legs, but it was minimal. "We are going to go through maneuvers that are standard after servicing—rolls

and accelerations and dives—through each of these, just keep
your eyes on the instruments, which will always tell you where
we are. The main ones in front of you are the altimeter—the
level will orient you to where you are as you cannot see over
my body. And then there is the speedometer to give you a
sense of how fast we are going. You can see only out the sides
and over through the top of the canopy." The voice, although
muffled and in Hebrew, made perfect sense to me.

"After my run in, I am going to do some low-level flying
and then some major climbs, which will really put your G-suit
and anti-G exercises to the test. If you do not feel well, let me
know. I will check with you every few moments to make sure
you have not passed out! We will fly up the old railway line
tracks to Jerusalem and then climb over Jerusalem. I have to
start my climb before we reach the city limits because of the
noise. It will be very low level for a while, with lots of back
and forth curving to keep with the changing landscape."

We rolled and ascended and descended in a way that I
could easily deal with. I even began to anticipate the way the
instruments would change as we moved. They would confirm
or counter my bodily feelings, which, often, could be out
of sync with what was happening when the G-suit started
increasing its pressure as we rapidly changed direction.

"Here we go to Jerusalem," Eitan said as we rolled
away from the center of the country. I could recognize the
landscape when I could see out of the sides of the canopy. It
kept changing, and I had to move my head from side to side
to see where we were headed. I could see from the altimeter
that we were pretty low—at most, hundreds of feet—and the
foliage was becoming greener in appearance and the trees
more plentiful. We rolled back and forth as we ascended
toward Jerusalem. I could see the world zooming past, too fast
for me to appreciate any landmarks.

"Ready?" he asked. "We will start our climb now—

your G-suit will inflate, and you must do your breathing maneuvers—this will take about thirty or forty seconds."

I could feel the tightening around my legs, and my abdomen began to be sucked into the back of me. I took a deep breath and started breathing out slowly, but with a grunting sound against my closed mouth, as I had learned in the course. The pressure was enormous; the altimeter was spinning madly around at, what seemed to me, hundreds of feet a second.

"Are you okay?" I could hear Eitan's somewhat muffled voice behind the roar.

I literally grunted with my Valsalva, "Yes!"

"We have a bit to go, and, when I get to 35,000 feet, we are going to roll over backwards, so look through the top of the canopy."

I wasn't sure how much longer I could hang on, so I focused on the altimeter: 9,000, 11,000, 15,000, 18,000, 25,000, 30,000, 35,000 ... Finally, the altimeter started to slow down and, with a feeling like nothing I had ever experienced in my life, at 35,000 feet, we looped over backwards, in a very wide circle. I could see the whole region spread out like a map— the Dead Sea, the Red Sea, the Kinneret (Sea of Galilee), the Mediterranean—and, as we started to descend, way down— like a small nugget—the glinting, gold Dome of the Rock in the middle of Jerusalem, whose ancient walls from here looked like a fine thread. The pressure dropped in the G-suit, and I could breathe easier. We leveled off, flew over the Negev, and started back to Hatzor.

Finally, we landed—the chute opening up the back of the plane to slow us down. They were all waiting for me—the clinic crew, some of the ground crew I had known over the years as patients and members of the base, even a few of the pilots who were my neighbors on the living compound. They applauded as I stepped down, and Eitan gave me a big handshake and a hug. "Not one drop of vomit!" he exclaimed. "A few more times and you can be my navigator."

*   *   *

We moved to Jerusalem two weeks later. Just before leaving, I handed in my gear, but kept my *sarbal* (flight suit), which they agreed to give me. The apartment was ready: I had purchased all the baby stuff for Neta the day after her birth as it was considered bad luck to furnish a baby's room before birth—the woman in the store knew all about that. Within two hours, everything had been loaded into the Saab to be delivered home, where I had assembled the crib so that all was ready for our homecoming. Yael's sister Daniela and Yael's mother, Chava, were there to help so that, by the night of our arrival, it really felt like we were "home."

A week later I reported to Shaare Zedek Hospital and spoke to the chief, Professor Jacob Menczel, and the two senior staff physicians. I was given a quick tour of the department and told to return on Sunday morning to start the job and meet the other house officers and residents. I was to be a senior resident, and would run a medical ward with three interns reporting to me.

Time passed. My Hebrew improved. I felt my competence as a physician grow. I found that I could run a busy emergency ward and a busy intensive care unit like a choreographer directing a dance group. In the middle of my first year, I returned for my first air force reserve duty—it was only four weeks—and, with the lull after the cease-fire from the War of Attrition, I spent my time at Tel Nof, another major air base in Israel proper, with two weekends on a forward air base— Refidim (Bir Gafgafa) in the Sinai Peninsula, where, in the past, I had done rotating weekends when I was stationed at Hatzor.

It was fairly quiet. The only memorable evacuation was that of a young Bedouin boy with severe measles and dehydration from Santa Katerina, a Greek Orthodox monastery in the Sinai Peninsula (said to be the place where the story of Moses and the burning bush occurred). The call came to Tel Nof and, because I always loved flying, I volunteered to go.

It was late afternoon when we left, and we were flying west as the sun began to set. The colors were magnificent. We could see the mountain and the monastery in the distance and white smoke coming from the helicopter landing area. The call had come from within the monastery, but the boy, his father, and a local nurse were waiting for us at the foot of the mountain. The boy was delirious, covered with a red, almost confluent rash, and he was very dry. The district nurse explained that the boy had been sick for four days and had not been eating or drinking for two. After speaking with the pilot, I explained to the boy's father, through the nurse as translator, that we were going to airlift him to a hospital in Israel and, in the meanwhile, would put an intravenous into him and give him fluids. The father asked some questions and received some answers. The nurse apparently told him that his son could die if we did not do this. He nodded in consent, and I inserted an intravenous line, which was not easy because of the boy's severe dehydration and resulting collapsed veins. The boy hardly budged, even when the needle pierced the skin. I ran the normal saline as fast as I could.

We loaded the boy in the Bell Huey helicopter, and the two medics fastened him in securely. The father was helped in next; he sat next to his son, almost kneeling beside him. The pilot told me that we were instructed to take him to Eilat, somewhat over an hour's flight away. As we lifted off with the gut-wrenching pull I had learned to love, I could see the wide-eyed look on the father's face as he stared out the glass on the doors watching the ground disappear and the monastery become a distant vision. We leveled off for the flight with the recurrent thump-thump of the rotating blades making it hard to hear. The IV was running well: the first liter was finished before we arrived, so I hung a second bag. I could see the lights of Eilat in the distance. The stars were bright outside without competing lights as we flew over the Negev.

Akaba was in the distance to the left of Eilat from the air, with fewer lights but an easy marker from anywhere around the Gulf. We could see the flashing lights of the helipad of the hospital and the white markings outlining where we were to land. The crew was there waiting with a wheeled stretcher. I had been recording the vitals on a clipboard—a liter and a quarter in; pulse down from 120 to 100 a minute; blood pressure still low—but the boy was now moaning and he fluttered his eyes when his father called his name. "*Salem Aleykum*," I yelled to the father as he jumped off the helicopter and ran after the wheeled stretcher—peace be with you. He turned back and smiled and waved his hand as he mouthed the words in return to me. We called the next day to hear that the boy had awakened that night after he received his third liter of fluids, was feeling much better, and was eating breakfast as we spoke.

It was during my last reserve duty that I had my first real experience of evacuation under fire. It was a pivotal experience in many ways as this was to be my last reserve duty before leaving the country to go to Canada for postgraduate medical training. The move to Canada had been a difficult decision, but, after long deliberations, Yael and I decided that it would be a good break from the pressures of Israel. Besides, the field of nuclear medicine, my intended area of study, was a specialty that did not exist in Israel. Yael was going to complete a PhD. We decided on Toronto because some colleagues I knew in Israel convinced us that it was a great city.

I hoped that, like my previous reserve duty, this would be a quiet time. The first days on the base were spent playing checkers, backgammon, and tennis, the latter being quite a challenge in flight suits and combat boots. One afternoon, while connecting with a tennis ball, my *hovesh* and I were summoned to the clinic, where I saw blood for transfusions being packed. We left shortly for a northern air base, fully loaded for medical evacuation with a flight crew, a *hovesh*, and two paratroopers on board. Our mission was to support the bulldozing of an east-west patrol road just below the Lebanese border, with perhaps some areas of minimal incursion across the border. Although the plan was a "peaceful" one, we knew that the Lebanese army might respond with armed intervention. We packed into our helicopter at five o'clock in the morning, eating our breakfast on the run.

There was room in the Huey for two evacuees at best. Whatever might have to be done to a wounded soldier also had to be done on the ground because the chopper's shaking precluded any medical intervention beyond basic maintenance. We flew north, the sun rising in the east. We were low off the ground. The sweet smell from budding almond trees wafted up from the orchards. From the open side door, I could see sleepy villages. We landed at a kibbutz near the Lebanese border.

The huge, dirty, bulldozers, covered in yellow armor, slowly gouged the road out of the hillside. Our first task after arriving at the kibbutz was to drop thousands of leaflets above dozens of villages in the vicinity. It seemed like a quiet, children's game with the only sound that of the helicopters going back and forth. We could hear gunfire in the distance and knew that there was some resistance. Paratroopers and infantry had gone in to intercept Lebanese soldiers who might be moving toward the bulldozers. Ground attack aircraft also flew some sorties, targeting some tanks that were moving in the direction of the border.

Suddenly the radio screeched: "Evacuation behind the lines!"

We bounded to the helicopter and, within moments, lifted off with that thrill of moving in three directions at once. In the distance we could see a couple of burned-out tanks—and then some running troops. We hovered a distance from a wounded soldier who was lying on a stretcher. We waited for the signal that it was safe to land nearby. As my *hovesh* and I arrived at the soldier's side, the pilot started signaling to take off immediately.

"Where are you injured?" I screamed at the soldier, trying to make myself heard above the roar of the engine. He grimaced and pointed to his back. There was no penetrating wound, but some bleeding, scrapes, and the back of his shirt was shredded a bit, as one might find in a fall. He said he could move his legs. We rushed to the helicopter and literally lifted off as we pushed in the stretcher, just barely managing to jump in ourselves.

We flew toward Haifa. I screamed at the patient, trying to make myself heard above the din of the engine and rotating blades. "Can you move your toes, legs, feel me pinching you?" I was able to elicit normal sensation on his legs above his combat boots, and I wondered just how severe the injury was. Could I be missing something more serious than what appeared to be the case? In the confines of the helicopter, it was impossible to properly examine him. I made sure he was secure in the stretcher and figured we would arrive at Rambam Hospital in about fifteen minutes as we were just flying south down the coast. Then I heard the captain through my earphones.

"How is your wounded soldier?"

"Stable," I answered.

"Any risk for further injury?"

"Why?" I asked.

"We have another soldier to evacuate—are we safe to go back?"

My heart dropped a beat. I was already picturing Haifa with its lovely harbor. On the other hand, the soldier seemed fine. I did not think I was missing a serious back injury that could lead to paralysis if we did not take him directly to hospital. There was another soldier needing evacuation, and we were clearly going to be the fastest to pick him up; otherwise, they would not have called us. The other medivac choppers must have been busy. My *hovesh* looked at me with anticipation. I signaled that our soldier was okay, so the *hovesh* tapped the pilot, indicating that we could return to the battle zone. The chopper made a tight turn—the kind I loved in general, but I didn't love that one so much, as I knew we were going into another potentially precarious situation.

The second soldier was sitting and waiting for us. He had a very bloody arm, already bandaged by an infantry *hovesh* on the ground. He looked pale and was in a lot of pain, although he had already been given some morphine. He did not have an intravenous running. I felt I had to put one in before we took off so I could give him blood en route. The pilot was frantically signaling that we had to leave, his hand circling over his head. I gave him the two-minute sign, and he frowned, but, for this, I was in charge. My *hovesh* had the tourniquet on in a moment, and I thrust in the Intracath™ with one smooth motion. As the blood rushed back, we taped the catheter securely, hung the saline, and the three of us ran to the chopper. Once there, the *hovesh* and I had to partially pick him up to get him through the door of the chopper, which was already hovering above the ground poised for takeoff. With the other soldier on the stretcher, it was tight inside. The chopper climbed very steeply, veering away from the combat zone. The fighting was drowned out by the sound of the engine. The soldier's pulse was rapid; we had to find a way to lay him down. We adjusted the other stretcher so that we could put the second one in place. Once he was comfortably placed, we partially removed the bandages and applied clean ones, making sure the pressure was such that it would halt any further bleeding which, clearly, had been quite severe. I hung a unit of O-negative blood and gave him some more morphine. Within five minutes, he seemed to settle down to the jostling lullaby of the chopper as, once again, we sped toward Haifa, the sun already beginning to lower itself over the Mediterranean.

Through the door and the cockpit windows, I could see the sea looming up on the right as, half-sitting and half-standing, I made sure the blood went through without problems. The soldier's pulse was steady, but there was no way to measure his blood pressure with the noise. I saw the helipad looming up at the top of the new Rambam Hospital, next to the one where I had worked as a medical student in 1965 and as an intern in 1967. We landed, and a crew of doctors and nurses immediately took the soldiers and transferred them to wheeled stretchers. Our mission accomplished, we lifted off again. The pilot turned and gave me the thumbs up. We heard later from the hospital that both of the evacuees were fine, and, though the second one required extensive surgery, he would not lose his arm. It was my last action of my last reserve duty.

The next month we left for Toronto, Canada, with our two children in tow.

Chapter 9

Shaare Zedek (Gates of Justice) Hospital

I was told that I should apply to Shaare Zedek for my medical residency, rather than Hadassah. "It is a very warm and friendly hospital, much smaller than Hadassah, with a very good teaching staff." I had heard similar comments from a few of the doctors I met during my military duties. So, I applied and was interviewed about six months before my tour of duty at Hatzor was to come to an end. Shaare Zedek was a very old hospital, situated at the entrance to Jerusalem on Jaffa road. Its primarily large wards reminded me a bit of the hospitals in Scotland, but it had a bit of a chaotic feel about it.

I was interviewed by Professor Menczel and Dr. Jacobson, the latter being an American gastroenterologist and one of the senior attending physicians on the internal medicine service to which I was applying.

"You will have a very good experience here. As you might know, we are a religious hospital, which sets us apart from some of the other hospitals. We do our best to follow Jewish law and its tenets of healthcare. We are affiliated with the Hebrew University, so are a real teaching hospital with medical students and postgraduate trainees assigned to us for their various clinical rotations. Most important for us, we have a reputation of being 'the hospital with a heart,' which is what you will see if you come and work with us. Also, we are small, so everyone really gets to know everyone else. You will not be lost as often happens in some of the other hospitals in Jerusalem."

This last bit was, clearly, a snide remark about Hadassah, the other main, very modern, and world-famous teaching hospital in the city.

I was able to take on the position of senior medical resident based on my previous training of almost two years of internships and a junior residency in Montreal. This meant I would be in charge of a medical team with three interns, myself, and the staff physicians. If there were medical students assigned to the service, they would be attached to our team as well—it was pretty much the same system I had experienced in Scotland, Boston, and Montreal. It was a busy place—busier than any hospital I had ever worked in, other than the city hospital in Athens, where I had gone as a medical student. I had never worked in a large American inner-city hospital, but expected that Shaare Zedek could compete with any of them for volume, severity of patient condition, and the feeling, at times, of utter chaos. The emergency ward was like a war zone. I had not quite realized when I took the position that once every fourth or fifth night and weekend (in essence, Friday night or Saturday in Israel), I would be the senior emergency room doctor, since the regular emergency physician signed over to one of us at 5:00 PM weekdays and on Friday nights until 8:00 AM Sunday morning (which, in Israel, is a regular workday).

During the two years that I was there—with a deduction of more than two months' military reserve duty, which was counted as part of the medicine rotational requirements—I spent almost six months starting up, and then running, an intensive care unit, followed by three months running the newly formed geriatric unit. I spent the rest of the time in general internal medicine. We did not have the luxury of medical subspecialty units or programs—everything was mixed up on the wards—so making rounds with the medical specialists was sometimes chaotic. Not knowing which patient was located where, we went from room to room looking for the patient about whom we were being consulted.

My Hebrew improved, but I could still not write in Hebrew and got permission, like a few of the other expatriate "Anglo-Saxons"—as we were referred to by the local Israelis or *Sabras*—to write my notes in English. I tried to master some Hebrew, but, at times, my notes became a mishmash of Hebrew and English blended together. In fact, once, after a long night on call, I found myself writing in English characters, but going from right to left! In addition to covering our medical wards, we rotated through the external medical consultation service for the hospital, which meant seeing patients on surgery, orthopedics, obstetrics and gynecology, and ophthalmology. This made life extremely busy, but served as an outstanding medical experience for my future career.

*   *   *

"It is getting close to the end," Dr. Jacobson said to me, speaking quietly, away from the patient who was in the emergency room with later stages of amyotrophic lateral sclerosis—Lou Gehrig's disease. The man in question was an Orthodox Jew who lived not far from the hospital in the ultra-Orthodox Mea Shearim district of the city.

"We have been using a cuirass respirator for a couple of months, which has helped a bit, but he is now mostly hypoxic (the tissues in his body were not receiving enough oxygen). We have to bring him in and see what we can do." (A cuirass respirator fits over the patient like a breastplate and aids the breathing.)

We spoke to Menczel, who was the most senior and experienced of the doctors, and Dr. Michael Goldstein, our respirologist from the States.

"Not much to do, really!" Goldstein said.

Menczel mused, "You know, when we had this type of respiratory muscular collapse during the polio epidemic in the fifties, we used iron lungs. I seem to think we still have one of the old machines somewhere in the basement. I wonder if we could use it."

He yelled out to Shmuel, the hospital's fix-it person. "Shmuel, do you remember the old iron lung? It was taken out some years ago when there was an exhibit of medical advances. Did we not put it back down in the basement somewhere?"

Shmuel laughed. "Sure. I know where it is; it is way in the back behind some of the old operating tables that we replaced. You know we never throw anything out in this place," he said, as he looked at me and winked. An hour later he and an orderly were wheeling in a yellow-colored steel contraption that looked like a miniature submarine, only with windows on the sides.

"It's like the yellow submarine from the Beetles!" I jokingly said. Shmuel started dusting it off and wiping it down.

"It will need some work if we are going to be able to use it. I have to check the rubber seals—some of them are probably cracked—and will have to fashion new ones in the shop, as there certainly won't be any parts for this. I also have to make sure the motor is working so it does not short out when we start it up. You would not want to put anyone in this thing unless it is working, right?"

In the meanwhile, we were keeping the patient breathing with a combination of the cuirass respirator and a re-breathing mask; it was not ideal, and we were ready to consider intubation if things turned sour. We explained to him what we hoped to do, to which he said, "Please send a note to my rabbi to ask what I should do. I do not know." Jacobson, whose written Hebrew was pretty good, wrote the note and the patient's brother, who also understood what we were proposing, took it and ran to Mea Shearim. He was back an hour later—and not too soon—as we already had been forced to start using an Ambu™ bag (a handheld device used to artificially ventilate a patient and often used in resuscitation) on the patient to keep his oxygen levels up. We did not want to intubate him unless we had the go-ahead from the rabbi to try the iron lung; after all, it was a real long shot. The answer was short— "Yes—whatever you can to save a life ... the ultimate duty of the physician—and of the patient—is to save his life."

We intubated the patient and attached him to our respirator in the ICU. He was awake, but lightly sedated. We waited while Shmuel worked on the yellow submarine all evening and into the night and then again in the early morning hours.

"I think it is ready to use, but we should really try it out," Shmuel said, as he and the orderly wheeled it into the large corridor between the medical ward and the geriatric ward— the only space large enough to hold it (we didn't think we should push it into the ICU unless we were actually going to use it).

"Right, we have to try it out," Menczel said, as he turned and looked at me with the familiar look that I knew would be followed by, "Michael, get into it!" Of course, he said it with his special Menczel smile. The two interns and Shmuel carefully opened the top of the machine and put me in after I had removed my clothes and put on hospital pajama pants and a T-shirt. It was tight as they closed the upper cover and secured the seal around my neck.

"Are you ready?"

"As ready as I'll ever be," I replied, as I heard the motor beginning to whir. Then, all of a sudden, I felt the wind being pulled out of me by a sudden negative pressure inside the submarine. I could not talk but could feel air being pulled into my lungs. A few moments later, the pressure left; I could exhale and said, "Wow!" and then it happened again.

I stopped trying to talk, allowing the machine to do its work. Shmuel played with the dials and sped up or slowed down the intervals until the machine—and I—reached a comfortable, "natural," steady state.

After five minutes, he shut it off, and I said to Menczel, "Let's go—it works—it's not easy, but it did not take long to get used to it."

We moved the machine into the ICU next to the patient and explained to him what we were going to do. As we disconnected him from the respirator, I bagged him until we could lift him into the submarine. We closed the seals, connected all the tubing, and Shmuel switched on the motor. A moment later, the negative pressure dial moved left below zero, and we could see the patient's inspiration (intake of air). Within ten minutes, he had achieved a rhythm, and, between cycles, was able to verbalize that he felt okay. After fifteen minutes, we performed a blood gas analysis, which came back normal.

"We did it!" I said to Menzcel.

We arranged for his place in the ICU, wrote out the orders for the nursing staff, and gave them a quick in-service as to how everything worked. We realized we would have to figure out how to feed him and take care of his need to urinate and defecate, but figured we had a bit of time to work out the particulars. In the interim, we arranged to take him out of the machine and bag him while putting him on a commode, and this arrangement worked the few times we tried it.

My beeper was sending out an urgent tone, and the overhead pager was calling my name to the ICU—dehoof (urgently). The patient was blue. He had aspirated some vomit that came up after a meal, another of the big challenges for us.

We were considering a permanent nasogastric tube, but felt that was an uncomfortable alternative. We tried suctioning him, and pulled him out of the submarine for CPR, but clearly it was a lost cause. I called off the *arrest*—resuscitation attempt—and pronounced him dead. A close friend of the family was outside the ICU; there was always someone from the family or community with him.

"We could not save him. Please go and tell the family."

The whole staff felt terrible, even though we knew it had been a long shot from the beginning. We shut off the submarine's motor, and the next day we sent it back down to the basement—maybe never to be used again. At least it was not used during the rest of my residency at the hospital.

*   *   *

Covering obstetrics was something I dreaded. When general medicine was called in, it was always bad news as the obstetricians and gynecologists, along with the anesthetists, could take care of anything else very well. The call came late in the afternoon; the ward was close to medicine so it was not a far run. As I rapidly approached the case room, I could see a man sitting outside, who I guessed was the husband. Inside, there were lots of people hovering over the patient, a young woman who was bleeding from everywhere.

"We have two units of whole blood hanging. She started bleeding and would not stop. We think the baby is dead, but now she is hypotensive (has low blood pressure). We sent blood off for more cross matching, but, in the meanwhile, we are giving her O-negative."

I noticed, as I raced around the bed and stepped in puddles of blood on the floor, that the blood was not very sticky.

"I think she has DIC—disseminated intravascular coagulation—maybe from an amniotic fluid embolism—very bad news. Get some fresh frozen plasma—we can try that."

As I called out that order, the nurse also called, "I think she has arrested!" The young mother was hooked to a monitor that showed a few complexes, then a straight line, and then a few complexes again.

"Call the arrest team!" I barked.

Twenty minutes later, with all of us covered in blood, we stopped the code, knowing it had been futile from the beginning. The obstetrician said, "I have to tell the husband. He is outside; he knew things were not good, but I don't think he realized how bad they were." I went with him as he broke the dreadful news to the man that he had not only lost his child, to have been his firstborn, but also his wife.

The howl and weeping were heart piercing. I went to the change room, removed my bloodied white coat, and took a very long shower before getting dressed again and returning to the medical ward.

*   *   *

"This is an interesting finding. Amantadine, a drug found helpful against contracting influenza, is also useful in patients with Parkinson's disease," noted Dr. Herishanu, the neurologist, while doing rounds on the geriatric unit where I was the resident in charge. L-dopa (L-3, 4-dihydroxyphenylalanine) had recently been released but already, we found that very few patients were able to tolerate it because of the severe gastro-intestinal side effects. They vomited their guts out and, after a few doses—even though their movements improved—would not take any more pills.

"We are going to try it on a few of our long-standing, most immobilized cases who are unable to tolerate the L-dopa."

I was skeptical. I had seen a few of the patients vomit after the L-dopa, and one man, in particular, was so immobile and heavy that it was very hard to move him. He had been bed and chair bound for over a year as the disease had progressed.

He was seventy years old and was waiting to move from the geriatric unit, where he had been admitted to try the L-dopa, to a situation in a nursing home that had recently become available. But nothing ventured, nothing gained … so we tried a course of Amantadine therapy.

The nurse called me over. "He is talking and moving."

I could not believe it. The patient had been receiving the medication for five days, receiving the full dose only on the past two days. I went to see the patient and, indeed, his face was mobile rather than fixed with the usual stare, and he was moving his legs and arms. We continued the drug, and, over the next few days, the physiotherapist started trying to get him out of the chair, which now had become possible. Within a few weeks, he could walk between parallel bars and with the help of a walking aid. He was delighted and was speaking. The staff was equally ecstatic, and Dr. Herishanu was very impressed.

"This is one of the best responses I have had, but we have treated only a few patients—this one is the first one here at the hospital. There are a few in my outpatient clinic who have just begun treatment, and they seem to be doing well so far. But these results are dramatic!"

Later, I was doing rounds when I heard a commotion from the physiotherapy gym. I rushed in to find the patient on the floor.

"He lunged at the medicine ball! We were doing exercises—he was doing so well and became excited with the game," said the physiotherapist.

From the clinical appearance, the area of pain, and the positioning of the leg, it was evident that he had fractured his hip. Surgery was performed, but the patient had a very bad postoperative course, and, less than a week after his surgery, he died very suddenly, we surmised from a pulmonary embolism.

*   *   *

Soon after, we had a case on the geriatric unit with a humorous flavor that counteracted the tragedy of the broken hip. I heard shouting in the dining room and ran there to find the staff standing around a patient of mine who had rheumatoid arthritis. They were yelling at him as they pulled his lunch plate from him, which he, in turn, was fiercely trying to get back. The patient was an elderly Iranian professor of Middle Eastern languages who spoke no English or Hebrew. He had been brought to the hospital through a series of errors the week before.

When he was brought in, I had been on call in the emergency department. Esther Cohen, a beautiful and very talented emergency room nurse of Indian-Jewish extraction of the *Bene Israel* (Sons of Israel) sect, had read the patient's history to me as I walked over to the stretcher in what had become a very crowded emergency room, not unusual for a Friday night when literally all the city's physicians signed out to the on-call service. Sending patients to the emergency room was very common with Saturday looming ahead.

"He is from Tehran and came to Israel via London, England, having been referred to Dr. Bloomberg, the rheumatologist at Hadassah Hospital," continued Esther. "They arrived this morning, and the taxi took them directly to the Hadassah emergency room. For some reason, the triage nurse did not realize that they were there because of a referral to a specific physician, and, since Hadassah is not on call today and we are, she sent him over to us. Now that it is after 5:00 PM, it will be impossible to contact Dr. Bloomberg's office until Sunday. So here he is. He has a four-month history of severe joint pain, especially in his hands and feet, as well as some generalized fatigue, weight loss with loss of appetite, and occasional low-grade fever."

"Do we have any blood work yet?" I asked.

"He has a mild anemia, but his renal (kidney) function seems okay, as are his lytes (electrolytes). That is all we have so far. His sedimentation rate is still being measured, and the rheumatoid factor will not be back until Monday or Tuesday."

Standing next to the patient, who was in his mid-sixties, was a woman in her early thirties.

"Do you speak English? How are you related to the patient?" I asked in English.

"I speak very little English but speak French—do you speak French?" she asked.

I answered her in my adequate, if not grammatically correct, French. She informed me that she was his daughter, and then related the history that the nurse had given. They had originally given the history in Farsi through a translator (we had a number of people working in the hospital originally from Iran). The nurse said the two had been happily surprised when they spoke to the translator. The patient told his daughter to tell us that he knew that many Iranian Jews had left their country, but did not realize that there were so many in Israel. This immigration phenomenon was explained to them by the translator who was, herself, originally from Tehran.

The daughter continued in French, "I am a nurse back home, but work in a neonatal unit. He began to feel unwell more than four months ago and went from one doctor to another and was prescribed various medications. We went to a big doctor in London who charged us a lot of money, but Father still did not feel better. A friend in Tehran—a professor at the medical school—told us about Dr. Bloomberg, and we arranged for an appointment. Father still feels awful."

I telephoned the staff physician on call and told him the story. "It sure looks like rheumatoid arthritis to me. He has not been given any reasonable dose of aspirin as far as I can make out; he has been taking them on an as-needed basis. I want to put him on anti-inflammatory doses and see how he does. I have one problem, though. There are no beds in medicine, and I just can't see putting him in the corridor—he is a 'visitor.'"

"What about the geriatric unit? We have a bed." Since I was the unit's resident, it was my call, and we arranged the transfer, with an order to administer nine hundred and seventy-five milligrams of aspirin four times a day, adjust the dose based on his joint pain and other symptoms, and watch for tinnitus (ringing in the ears—a sign that we were giving him too much). In that case, we would have to pull back a bit. By about 10:00 PM that night, he had been moved to the geriatric unit and had already received one dose of aspirin, with another to be given two hours later.

I started making rounds on the geriatric unit at 9:00 AM the next morning, after having been up most of the night with the emergency room coverage. It was a tiring routine, but pretty standard in those days. I entered a four-bed room, which was considered almost luxurious compared to the larger eight- and twelve-bed rooms on the general medical ward. The patient was in the bed near the window. I asked the nurse if she could find a particular member of the dietary staff, whom I knew spoke Farsi. Five minutes later, Batya came in, and we walked over to the patient.

"How are you today?" she asked on my behalf.

Before he could say anything, I could see by the way he was holding his hands that they were less painful.

"A bit better—not as much pain this morning—thank you."

"Ask him if he has any ringing in his ears," I said to her.

He answered that he did not, and, when I touched his swollen hand joints, they seemed a bit less inflamed than they had been the night before. But it was still less than twelve hours into treatment. Over the next few days, he continued to improve, but, on the fifth day, he said his ears were ringing a bit, so we cut back on his aspirin dose. We discussed switching him to the newly released anti-inflammatory drug, Ibuprofen, but it was much more expensive than the aspirin we were using. Also, we didn't stock Ibuprofen at the hospital.

It was on his sixth day with us that the event in the dining room occurred. His daughter had brought him in some yogurt, which he loved. Prior to this, both of them had received an explanation of the hospital's kosher food rules. Unfortunately, the patient did not realize that pouring the yogurt over the sliced beef that had been brought to him for lunch was not acceptable in a strictly kosher environment, and this was why everyone was yelling at him and trying to pull his plate away. We settled the misunderstanding, with apologies extended by everyone.

Given that he was only being prescribed aspirin, was improving, and was now able to walk around, we agreed that he could return to the King David Hotel. He and his daughter had a large room there, and it was agreed that I would visit him there on my way home from work. I did this for the next few days, but he had clearly improved and wanted to go home.

I came by the day before he was going to return home via London (as there were no direct flights from Israel to Tehran for political reasons). His daughter said to me, "My father is very grateful for everything you have done for him. He would like to give you a gift. Would you like some English cloth for a suit? He knows a wonderful tailor in London."

I smiled and said, "In Israel, I would have no use for a suit. No one wears them here, so, no, thank you, but that is very kind. It is not necessary."

She explained to her father, and then, after a moment, said, "How about if we sent you a Persian carpet from home? They are very beautiful."

"Really, that is not necessary. I probably could not even afford the import tax on a carpet on the salary that I make, and our apartment is not large. I do not think we could use a carpet."

She went into the bedroom—the suite had two rooms—

and came out a few moments later with a gift-wrapped box. "Here is a small token of our appreciation. It is some sweets, which I think you and your family will like."

I thanked the two of them very much and gave them a letter with a summary of his hospital stay for his doctor in Tehran. In turn, they gave me their address and invited me to visit, which I knew would be very unlikely in those days even though, at the time, Israel had relations with the country, which was then under the shah's rule.

Some weeks later, one evening, I decided to open up the box of sweets, wondering if they might be too rich for our taste. As I took off the wrapper, an envelope fell out in which I found a thank-you letter and $500 in U.S. currency, an amount of money equal to three months of my salary. I was overwhelmed.

We left a few weeks later for Toronto so that I could embark on a career in nuclear medicine. With two children—one, just having turned two, and the other three months old—we left the country with the assumption that we would return in two to three years. It would never happen.

Chapter 10

The Wonders and Joys of Geriatrics

My first exposure to geriatrics came when I was a medical student in Dundee. The professor and registrar had figured among my favorite teachers, and the geriatric unit was a large ward with a potbellied stove in the middle that, during the evenings, warmed the patients who were able to sit around it. The ward had a very warm and inviting atmosphere. My geriatric experience in Israel was also special, and my time in the ward at Shaare Zedek Hospital was one of the highlights of that residency period. The confluence of opportunity and a chance meeting resulted in my making contact again with Dr. Abe Rapoport, whom I had met in Israel just prior to leaving for Toronto. After we discussed my options for further training, he suggested I contact Drs. Henry Himel and Cyril Gryfe at the Baycrest Centre for Geriatric Care in Toronto. I visited the centre, and, when Dr. Barney Berris offered me a chief residency position in medicine at Mt. Sinai Hospital, an institution with a strong connection to Baycrest, my fate was set.

Within weeks of providing consultations on the older

patients from Baycrest, or for whom Baycrest might be the discharge destination, I realized that I had finally found my place in medicine. After my chief residency and successful completion of the Royal College examinations in medicine in 1976, I was offered a conjoint position at both organizations. My career path was settled. With the establishment of the specialty of geriatric medicine at the Royal College in 1981— and my receipt of its first certificate—there was no turning back. For the next thirty years, the practice of geriatric medicine became my passion, providing me with both inspiration and professional satisfaction throughout my medical career at the two organizations, both of which were affiliated with the University of Toronto. Contrary to the negative biases held by many of my medical colleagues and members of the public, the field of geriatrics is neither depressing nor futile. In contrast, it is full of medical challenges and the great satisfaction of dealing with individuals who have had long, varied, and often very fascinating lives and experiences. The life story of the patient and how it may have contributed to current medical issues is a point I like to stress when teaching medical students and postgraduate medical trainees the diagnostic skills required in the care of the elderly.

*   *   *

He was very ill—semicomatose, with no focal neurological findings, yet not readily aroused. The team had asked me to see him as part of my teaching rounds. Despite the absence of neurological findings, the attending physicians had assumed the seventy-seven-year-old, previously healthy man had suffered a stroke. His blood pressure was up, and there were problems with his kidney function. As the group of interns and final-year medical students hovered around, listening and watching, the resident related the medical history to me. It was my second week as chief medical resident—and only my second real teaching case, the first having been a patient with pneumonia and heart failure, not a problem for me as I had seen many cases like this as senior and chief medical resident in Israel. However, this particular one was more of a challenge.

"He has a systolic ejection murmur, but no evidence of heart failure," said the final-year medical student who was responsible for presenting the case in response to my questions.

We went through the history, physical findings, and the laboratory results to date, and I started questioning the student, allowing additional input from the group. "What are these spots on his lower limbs and toes?" I asked, pointing to some bluish-reddened areas. Everyone looked.

"I had not noticed them and am really not sure," replied the student.

"What do you see in his retina?" I asked, thinking in terms of increased intracranial pressure, a possible cause of his semicomatose state. Again, there was a blank stare, and the student replied, "I could not see in his pupils and was afraid to dilate them because of his obtunded (semicomatose) state."

"Let's get in some drops with a short half-life so we can see what is going on with him," I suggested. A few moments later, the drops were instilled as we continued through the neurological examination. There were no abnormalities in the reflexes. The heart murmur was quite pronounced, which led to a discussion of the causes, which could have included aortic stenosis, or, most likely in a man of his age, sclerosis of the aortic valve. As the pupils dilated, I took out the ophthalmoscope and, even though the patient was on the bed farthest from the window and the curtain was closed, I asked one of the interns to dim the light in the room and another to close the window blinds. I wanted the room to be as dark as possible.

There they were: little yellow slits in the retina—

geometrically shaped—reflecting the light from the ophthalmoscope in a glinting manner. My heart raced as I realized I had made an obscure diagnosis. I looked in both eyes and confirmed my observation. "Here," I said, as I gave the ophthalmoscope to the student.

"I have not done that many of these before," he said as he started looking toward the eye.

"Keep the other eye open and start further back," I instructed, "and wait till you see the red reflex and follow it in. When you see the retina, focus carefully—yes, that's it. Now angle it up and down and tell us what you see."

"I can see the blood vessels; they do not seem abnormal. I do not see any hemorrhages … wait! I see something that looks yellow—I see two of them—but I am not sure what they are." He stood up and gave the ophthalmoscope to one of the interns, who more handily took the device and started looking.

"I see both of them too—and another—they are yellow and angular, like geometrical shapes, a bit shiny."

The medical resident took the ophthalmoscope. "Oh my goodness, I see them—like crystals, like gout in the eye—but that can't be! What kind of crystals can get into the eye?"

As we talked through the case, it became apparent to all that these were athero-embolic crystals made of cholesterol-containing material, which is why they looked shiny and had their particular shape. And, if they were in the eye, then they were likely in the brain. Given what we had seen in his feet and his poor kidney function, no doubt they were everywhere. His body had been showered with them. With the flow of blood from his abnormal aortic valve, in all likelihood, the crystals were washed into each organ, where they caused severe and likely permanent damage. As there was no treatment for the condition, we had little to offer other than the diagnosis and a poor prognosis.

I thanked the group for the very challenging and most

interesting case, and, as I walked away, I could hear the word "amazing" said repeatedly (which I hoped was being applied to me as well as to the patient we had just discussed). It seems that I had passed my first test among the house staff and students and would not have to prove myself again.

It was hard to believe that, only a few months before, I had not been sure I would ever get to this place. I had felt very self-conscious sitting with all the final-year students in the large auditorium for the beginning of a series of lectures that would prepare them for the licensing examinations before they became interns. I was a good deal older then most of them. While waiting for the lecturer to arrive, the person next to me asked, "So where are you going next year?" I turned and looked at the young face and replied, "Mt. Sinai Hospital, probably." "Really? Me, too! I'm doing a straight in medicine—what about you?"

I said with some hesitation in my voice, "Well, I'm supposed to be chief medical resident. So I might be seeing you."

"Oh, great—so why do you have to take this exam and attend these lectures? You must know it all—chief resident … wow!"

"I have been overseas for a while and did not study in Canada, so I need to take the exams and get licensed. This is just for some brushup."

Actually, another physician and I had been asked to share the role of chief medical resident. I had stretched the truth hoping that the student could not discern the nervousness I was feeling at the prospect of failing these exams and then not being able to take on the job. The lecture started, and I absorbed myself in a way I had not done for years—listening and taking notes—trying to place new concepts into a memory by now mixed with medical school education and years of clinical training, but not much didactic structure, which was what I had to get back over the next month if I were to pass the exam. I felt a modicum of terror as I copied the figures of the immune system that were displayed by the lecturer.

The fateful meeting with Dr. Abe Rapoport in Jerusalem that resulted in my being offered the chief residency position at Mt. Sinai was one event in a chain of events that, when I look back, seems to have been meant to be. The Yiddish and Hebrew term *beshert*, which reflects that concept, seemed to characterize the chain of events that led me to this year, one that turned out to be merely the prologue to a long and satisfying career in geriatrics.

My first year in Toronto had been dedicated to training in nuclear medicine, the program to which I had applied while in Israel, but it became clear early on that it was not a suitable career path for me. Nevertheless, I completed the year knowing that a commitment is a commitment, and that leaving in the middle of the year would not only be unfair to the department, but completely out of character for me. During that year, I also realized that the income from my residency would not be sufficient to maintain our family's living needs in Toronto. I was lucky to have someone recommend me for some moonlighting shifts at a local emergency room. Given my background in internal medicine in Israel—and the fact that I had run Jerusalem's Shaare Zedek Hospital's intensive care unit for almost six months while working almost every four days in one of Jerusalem's busiest emergency rooms—the moonlighting duties at the Northwestern Hospital seemed like a relative walk in the park. No less important, the money I made was fabulous compared to my regular salary, and made such a difference in our income that we were able to avoid the embarrassment of having to borrow money from my parents, something I definitely did not want to do.

The year as chief medical resident was very challenging and satisfying. I decided to prepare for the Royal College examinations in the fall. This meant that, in addition to everything else I had to do, I also needed to find time to study for a kind of examination that I was not all that used to, although recently I had tasted a flavor of the process when I had sat the licensing examinations. In addition to studying for my examinations, I also hoped to excel as much as I could in my chief residency role. I had much to learn about the Canadian healthcare system, which I enjoyed because it seemed much like the National Health Service where I had trained, and was quite unlike the system I had experienced in Boston. In Canada, thankfully, the financial or "insurance" status of a patient was not part of the patient-physician discussion. In fact, I never heard anyone tell me that something could not be done because a patient was not insured. Most importantly, I quickly found out how much I enjoyed dealing with the elderly Baycrest patients who, for the most part, had been given relatively short shrift by some of my colleagues, who welcomed my desire to take on their care. Over the next few months, as the examinations loomed and the study groups into which I had been accepted became more intense and focused, I became quite nervous about the outcome, especially since people were constantly asking me how things were going.

"Dr. Berris (which was how I addressed Barney out of deference and respect), I am not sure I can sit these exams right now. I just have too much on my plate, and so many people are asking about my studying. Maybe I should take them next spring instead."

"Michael, you can pass them. I know you can," he said. "But when people ask you how you are doing, why not just say you may not be taking them this time around and leave it at that? Eventually, they will stop asking and you will be able to focus as you feel more comfortable. If you don't think you can sit them at that point, then you don't have to, but I think you can breeze through them."

I took his advice, and, over the next few weeks, fewer and fewer people asked me about them. I advised the study group that I would continue to attend so I could keep up-to-date, but no longer revealed my intentions. On the day of the exams, I turned up—much to the surprise of some of my colleagues—but at this point they were into their own space, so it did not matter much. Three weeks later, the letter announcing my pass arrived. I gave Barney a great big hug and could not help but notice the warm smile on his face.

The oral examinations were to take place a month later. To help me prepare, Barney said, "Each time you present a patient to me that you have seen, let's work through the situation as if it is your oral." We did these mock runs week after week, and, when the time finally came, I took the train to Montreal and, along with other candidates from Toronto and elsewhere across the country, went through the cross-examination ritual, keeping Barney's words in the forefront of my consciousness: "Just do what you do with me every day." I did so, and, by the time I left the city, I had my answer and my fellowship in internal medicine.

Later that month, I was offered the position of my dreams: part-time at Mt. Sinai as an internist with a special interest in the care of the elderly, and part-time at Baycrest as one of the staff internists looking after the elderly population who lived, or were hospitalized, there. My future seemed to be set, and, with life seemingly more settled, I was able to focus more and make myself more available to my interns and residents for supervision and teaching. Within a week, I was confronted with a real clinical conundrum.

The patient was in his early sixties and bearded, as one might expect in the Orthodox community. In his cursory style, the resident told me the story: "Immigrant, eighteen years ago from Israel. Had been in reasonably good health. Developed a flu-like illness two weeks ago which lingered. Had headache about three days ago with increased fever. Family doctor gave him antibiotics, and last two days—very confused and feverish."

I inquired about the patient's past history. "Where was he before he lived in Israel?"

The resident seemed puzzled and looked to the clinical clerk who had done the admission. "I don't know. I just assumed he came from Israel. Why do you ask?"

I was always amazed at the contrast between the students and medical trainees in Scotland and other parts of the UK and Israel—places where I had completed most of my medical training—and those from Canada or, for that matter, the United States. When I studied, it would have been almost unheard of for a student to question a staff physician rather than just acknowledging his seniority and de facto superior knowledge and wisdom. Yet the question asked by the clinical clerk was in fact most appropriate, most welcome, and was key to my thinking. The answer was critical if we were to have any special insights into this patient and provide an important teaching point to the trainees.

"Many Israelis, in fact, came to Israel from Europe and, from the timing in your story, it is likely that he came from Europe. If this was after the war, it's quite possible that he was interned in a concentration camp. How might we check that out if there is no one to ask?" I asked. "The family members are not here, he is severely delirious and not really in a position to be answering questions right now."

The resident—a Canadian-born Jewish doctor—and the clinical clerk, who was not Jewish, and the two interns, who were Jewish, all looked at me.

"Roll up his left sleeve and let us see what is on his arm," I said. The telltale pale blue numbers were there—a bit faded—but a clear indication of where he had spent some years of his life.

"Concentration camp survivors often contracted tuberculosis in the camps and can still harbor the bacteria since they likely would not have received any treatment." I pulled his sleeve back down and put my hand behind his head and exerted pressure. His body moved forward, but his neck did not bend.

"Get a lumbar puncture tray. Let's look at his chest x-ray, if you did one already, and, if you didn't, let us get one as soon as possible."

The cerebrospinal fluid gave us the answer, as did the chest x-ray, which showed healed tubercular lesions. Protein levels were high; the glucose level on the low side, but within the normal range; and the laboratory reported that there were a few reddish bacilli on the special Ziehl-Nielsen stain, highly indicative of the diagnosis. I was worried about administering a tuberculosis test, but, after conferring with the infectious disease expert, we decided to do one while we started him on therapy. It was not easy to give the test to someone in his condition. Two days later, the red patch on his arm—a positive reaction to the TB test—was so angry looking that I was afraid it would break down, but, with treatment now underway, he was less drowsy and his fever was lower. As he improved, his wife, whom he had met in Israel—though not a Holocaust survivor—confirmed our initial assumption. She could not believe that now he might survive. She and her family had already assumed the disease was fatal.

Six weeks later, long after his clinical condition attested to our correct assumptions, the culture came back positive. He went home and was followed up in the infectious disease clinic with no further problems. Many years later, he was admitted to Baycrest following a severe stroke, and his wife reminded me how I——though I quickly corrected her to say "we"—had saved his life before and she hoped we could do it again. Sadly, now twenty years later, what he was suffering from, while not as life threatening as tuberculosis, would, unfortunately, not respond as dramatically to treatment. He spent the rest of his days at Baycrest with neurological impairment, but he and his wife always had a very warm greeting for me whenever I met them, she often pushing him in his wheelchair.

*   *   *

Those months between the time I passed my examinations and the time I took on my staff position were among the most illuminating of my career. During those months, I began to crystallize my understanding of the care needs of the elderly, years before Canada finally agreed to a certification in the field and the first examinations, which took place in 1981. I found that, since there were few mentors locally other than a few of the Baycrest physicians and a British physician from a nearby Veterans Administration Hospital, I had to draw on my experiences from Scotland and Israel where, at Shaare Zedek Hospital in Jerusalem, the first real geriatric unit in an acute care hospital had opened. Those experiences, coupled with my interest and curiosity, helped consolidate my own understanding of the aging process so that I might assist other physicians who expressed an interest in the field to achieve some degree of expertise and exposure.

I have long believed that there is an excessive focus on science education as the prerequisite for medical school. This has become more pronounced during the past few years. (In the United States students must satisfactorily complete pre-medical subjects in order to qualify for medical school, though this can be achieved within a context of a non-science major or a mixed education.) Over the years, I have found that my exposure to literature, classics, philosophy, and history had a far more important and sustained impact on my ability to practice medicine than the courses in chemistry, biology, and physics, which were part of the premedical requirements. In fact, the last time I looked at Krebs biochemical equations and cycle was in second-year physiology at medical school, but I continue to refer to my exposure to philosophy, history, and literature and, in my teaching activities, refer more often to these fields than the fields of pure science. It is not that science is not important to the preparation for and understanding of medicine, it is that the arts are also needed to promote intellectual and humanistic balance.

Having a background understanding of languages other than English has always been of benefit to me in life and, periodically, also in the practice of medicine. During my chief residency, I was often asked to review patients who were going to or coming from surgery because of medical problems, or to assess their suitability for institutional placement. (The staff had quickly learned that I was the medical connection to Baycrest and its long-term care, chronic care, and rehabilitation beds.) They really were not asking for an opinion because of my medical expertise (which, for many of my colleagues, appeared to be mysterious); they really were asking for referral—other than perioperative care—in order to free up an acute care bed by shuttling an older patient to Baycrest or some other long-term care institution.

One of these sorts of consultations came from the orthopedic service. It was for a patient I had not been asked to see prior to urgent hip surgery for a fracture she apparently had sustained in a fall at her apartment. The terms "demented and confused" were included in the assessment on the orthopedic admission notes; this seemed enough to foreclose any further investigation into her mental status or possibilities of rehabilitation. Her granddaughter had found her on the floor three days after she had last visited with her. By that time, the patient was quite dehydrated and confused, so the consent had come from the granddaughter, who then had to leave town on a business trip, and was, therefore, unavailable for me to interview.

I entered the room, already noting in the chart that the patient was classified as "demented and confused." This seemed to have been transcribed from the initial assessment by the orthopedic resident. When I asked for an update at the nursing station, they said the patient was constantly muttering "gibberish." I found a thin, elderly woman in bed, edentulous (without teeth). The side rails on the bed were up, presumably to keep her from climbing out of bed. There was a food tray by her bed. It was a bit far away for her to easily reach, so hardly anything had been eaten. I started to speak to her, slowly and distinctly, but not loudly, and she turned toward me.

"*Deutsche, kennen sie Deutsche?*" It was difficult to decipher because she had no teeth, but it sounded to me as if she wanted to know if I spoke German. My Yiddish knowledge and my years traveling through Europe brought forth from the recesses of my brain, "*Ya, kennen sie* English?"

"*Nein, nur Deutsche,*" which I knew meant she spoke only German. I continued in my broken Yiddish/German, "*Wie geht es Ihnen?*"(How are you?) She responded emphatically, "*Sehr schlecht. Ich habe chmerz und Ich bin hungrig.*" (Very bad; I have pain and I am hungry.) I told her that we would take care of everything and went back to the nursing station. "Does anyone here speak German or Yiddish?" The nurses looked at me with blank stares. "That patient, whom every one thinks is demented and confused, is neither," I informed them. "She speaks only German, and she says she has pain and is hungry. Is anyone attending to her or communicating with her?"

The head nurse overheard my conversation and came out and said, "Really? No one brought that up. We assumed she was out of it—you know she *is* ninety years old."

"That may be so," I replied, "but she was living at home, wasn't she? Isn't that where they found her? Did anyone take a detailed, functional history from the granddaughter?"

It took a few hours to locate a proper translator, place the patient on a pain regimen, move the food tray close to her, and arrange for someone from volunteer services to help feed her and start getting her out of bed and into a chair. The physiotherapist had been told there was no rehabilitation potential because she was demented. However, when she was able to communicate with the patient, she determined that the patient could follow directions, and so started her on a therapeutic program. I was, indeed, able to move her to Baycrest, but for rehabilitation, not the chronic care that had formed the basis of the original referral. When the granddaughter appeared some days later, she confirmed her grandmother's unilingualism, as well as the fact that the older woman managed to live on her own with assistance from the granddaughter perhaps a few times each week. And, when she brought in the grandmother's dentures from home (which she had failed to do when the ambulance arrived to take her to the hospital), the grandmother's speech became quite clear and understandable. The day before we were transferring her to Baycrest, I went to see her and wish her well. She took my hand and said, as clearly as anyone could ever want to hear, "*Vielen dank fur helfen mir.*" (Thank you for helping me.) To which I replied, "*Auf wiedersehen.*" (I will see you again, good-bye.) Three months later, she went home.

That was just one case in which assumptions had been made by attending physicians and nurses about the mental status of older patients who were not functioning well and who, then, were quickly labeled as demented and in need of chronic or long-term care. Since I was part of that conduit, over the years I saw many patients where the assumption concerning their mental status was incorrect, and, with the appropriate treatment, the outcome proved to be much better than anyone would have expected. So, with the diagnosis of dementia—or with patients who developed states of mental confusion postoperatively—the assumption was often that they "must have suffered a little stroke." This amorphous group of patients was the source of many of my referrals and served as the basis of my learning about the frailty of the older brain. I came to realize just how often older hospitalized patients were misdiagnosed and mislabeled. Once designated as such, it was very hard for the medical and nursing staff in charge of their care to change their mind-set with respect to what the diagnosis held for them: unsuitable for active treatment and simply in need of placement—but somewhere else—outside of the acute care hospital that was their domain.

*   *   *

Mrs. Fischman was eighty-seven years old and had lived with her daughter before being admitted to hospital with pneumonia. I had seen her a year previously when she needed and had benefited from the cataract surgery for which I provided the pre- and postoperative medical care. At that time, she had been functioning reasonably well and lived in an apartment with her daughter. But her treatment was taking a rocky course during this admission. Initially, she did not respond well to antibiotics, developing an infected pleural effusion (fluid in the lung cavity) and kidney problems due to the fluids and antibiotics she was receiving. Eventually, the infection cleared up, but she gradually stopped eating and lay in bed without communicating with anyone. I was asked to see her for placement at Baycrest with a diagnosis of severe dementia (known in those days as "organic brain syndrome"). Her daughter remained by her side almost all the time.

"I just do not understand," she said to me when I introduced myself and explained that I had been asked to arrange her transfer to Baycrest. "Until she got sick, she was okay. Although I did all the shopping and she only went out with me when the weather was nice, she seemed okay. She sometimes talked about how much of a burden she was to me, but I have been widowed for nine years, my children are all settled and only see us once in a while. I always told her that she was not a burden. She did so well after the eye surgery and was happy to be able to watch television again. And now this ... I just don't understand."

After looking through the health record, I could not find any explanation for her current state. They had even performed a CT scan, thinking she may have had a stroke, but there was no evidence of that; and her brain was not all that atrophied for a woman of her age. What I found intriguing when I examined her was that she was curled up on her left side, facing the bed rails, her eyes, for the most part, closed. She could open them when spoken to, but did not reply when asked questions. She didn't seem to acknowledge or recognize me, even though I had seen her several times during the previous cataract surgery hospitalization. She had stopped eating and now had a nasogastric feeding tube in place, which was clearly annoying her. She had developed some redness and inflammation around the nostril through which the tube was inserted. I thought she might be severely depressed and considered my options—one of which was to put anti-depressant medications through the feeding tube—but it could be weeks before she would respond to the drugs, and she might succumb by the time they would have an effect. I arranged to speak to the psychiatrist who had used "organic brain syndrome" as a diagnostic label.

"I think she is severely depressed … almost catatonic," I explained to him. "There is no other reasonable explanation. Her lab work and CT scan are all normal, and she was expressing depressive thoughts prior to becoming ill."

"I cannot get a history to confirm depression, and using ECT (electroconvulsive therapy) would be quite a bold step," he replied. "I am not sure I could take that risk—you know people feel very funny about it. And I could not get consent from her, of course."

"She is going to die this way—this is a real medical emergency," I responded. "I believe I can get consent from the daughter if I give her a full explanation of the urgency of this treatment—and all the risks. I would do it myself if I owned the machine, but I don't—you do. So I will take all the responsibility and will follow her—I just need you to do the treatments. Please, I need your help on this."

He looked a bit uncomfortable but said, "Okay, but I

will need you to record in the chart that you are taking the responsibility for this decision and will inform the daughter. Right?"

"Right!" I agreed. I spoke to the daughter frankly about why I thought we should do the ECT treatments, and advised her that it was only with great reluctance that the psychiatrist had agreed.

"I know she is going to die if we do not do this," said the daughter. "I don't want her to die. I agree to what you recommend."

The day after the third treatment, I entered the floor and one of the nurses said, "Your girlfriend is up in a chair." I turned the corner from the nursing station and there was Mrs. Fischman, sitting in a chair, with half a cheese sandwich and a glass of milk on her tray. "Dr. Gordon, how are you? Would you like something to eat?" She offered me the second half of her cheese sandwich. At this point, and before I could decline the offer, her daughter came out of her room and said, "Look at her, she is up and talking! They said it would take at least a week of treatments—this is just after three—can you believe it?"

I reviewed the record and saw that she had pulled the tube out the night before and asked for something to drink. Clearly this had been a most dramatic response. The psychiatrist left me a message that he would finish the course of treatments as planned and expressed satisfaction with the outcome. I thanked him. Mrs. Fischman was discharged three weeks later back to her home. The daughter sent me a note a few months later telling me that they decided to apply for a nursing home for her as she was feeling quite cooped up in the apartment and wanted to go someplace where there would be activities with others her age! Mrs. Fischman had expressed again that she did not want to be a burden to her daughter, but she was still eating and drinking, listening to music, and watching television, her main pastimes before her recent hospitalization.

*   *   *

In addition to my hospital practice, my office practice gradually began to grow. At one point, when I had a number of half-day offices open with no patients scheduled for consultation, I became a bit despondent, feeling that no one seemed to understand the importance of what I might contribute as a physician who focused on the care of the elderly. I considered expanding the practice to include general medicine. As he had done many times before, Dr. Berris gave me wise advice, "Don't do it. Sit it out. They will come. If you change the focus of your practice, you will have problems changing it back. And then you will be stuck—not able to do what you want to do. So, bring a book and wait. People will eventually recognize the value of what you provide, and they will come."

Dr. Berris must have consulted a magical crystal ball, for, within four months, my office was fully booked each week, with a waiting list that started moving a few weeks into the future. My geriatric clinic at Mt. Sinai Hospital was launched.

During this clinic experience, I began to really learn about geriatric medicine. What happened in the clinic was very different from anything I had experienced in the past in general internal medicine clinics. Here, there was not just a focus on diagnosis and treatment, but on the impact of illness on the family, as well as the social context of the person who was often beginning to fail. Dealing with these issues and helping patients, as well as their families, required a greater scope of engagement than I had been used to when practicing general medicine. As I continued to observe the patients and their families, my self-education expanded and began to fit within the totality of what was being taught and published. I found that my own observations were sometimes at odds with the current dogma; this served to further stimulate my academic curiosity. Many of my patient encounters were particularly satisfying, surprising, or held an element of poignancy that was almost unique to the practice I found myself developing.

One patient was sent to me with a likely diagnosis of Alzheimer's disease, but the family doctor was insecure about starting one of the newer treatments for it, given that the literature was somewhat ambivalent about the drug's effectiveness. He knew that I supported its use, despite the fact that many of my colleagues credited my positive views to an inherent optimism rather than substantial evidence of benefit shown in standard cognitive scores. Yet, I could not help but believe the families of the patients who often recounted important improvements with the medications, despite little evidence of real change in the scores of standard cognitive tests. Nor could I explain the disparity, other than to assume that the test may have been an inappropriate measurement tool, even though it had been one of the standards used in the drug evaluation process.

The patient and her husband were concerned because she was losing her abilities in English. German was her mother tongue, and she was reverting back to it more and more. She was especially experiencing difficulty reading books in English, which had been one of her favorite activities for the forty years she had been in Canada. During our initial meeting, we spent a great deal of time talking about literature—a favorite subject of mine—and, clearly, she was well read and able to discuss a wide array of books she had read in the past. Since I was familiar with many of them, I could attest to her knowledge of and fluency with them. It was newer literary challenges that were causing the problem: she said she had stopped reading the book review section of the newspaper many months before because the reviews no longer made that much sense, and she was unable to remember afterwards which books might be of interest to her.

After discussing the potential benefits and side effects of the various medications for cognition and the skepticism about them expressed by some observers, she eagerly agreed to try the medication. I gave her a prescription for the drug and arranged to see her for follow-up in three months. The week before I saw her, I had begun reading Guy Vanderhaeghe's novel *The Last Crossing*. By chance, the book had been reviewed in the book section of one of the local newspapers the weekend before my clinic. I had some problems getting into the book because of the number of characters. However, the characters become clarified as the book progresses and, already, I was becoming enthralled with the story. The book review commented on that very aspect of the book and encouraged readers to persevere because the quality of the book would make it worth their while. That clinic afternoon, the first-year family medicine resident working with me as usual examined the patient on my behalf before our review together. He came into my office, very excited. "She can't wait to see you! You are going to be very happy. I read your note, and I have never seen anything like this, though, granted, I have not seen many patients with Alzheimer's disease who have been put on this medication. Two months ago, my supervisor expressed doubt that the drug was really worth using and gave me an article from the United Kingdom to read that shed a very negative light on this whole class of drugs."

We entered the room together and there she was, sitting with her husband, patiently waiting to see me after having spent quite a while with the resident, who had readministered the mental status examination (it took him rather a long time because he had not yet done this very often in his training). The score was substantially higher than evidenced on the previous visit. I looked at the patient and, after the niceties of greetings had been exchanged, realized that this might be a "teachable moment" to demonstrate to the resident the importance of collateral support for impressions that are often outside the standard mental status measure. In my view, these are at least as—if not more—important. I looked at the patient, who was sitting next to her husband, a semiretired academic.

"So, have you been able to read anything in English?"

She nodded, "Yes."

"What have you been reading lately?" I asked.

She smiled and said, "Yes, last month I started reading again and have continued to do so."

"So what is your latest?"

"I started a book two weeks ago, which I found a bit hard to get into, but now I am actually beginning to enjoy the story. The writer has a long complicated name, Van der bilt—no, that is not it. Van der haven? No, but something like that; it's a bit of a funny name."

"Vanderhaeghe. Is that it?" I asked.

"Yes, that's it! A book about a crossing—*The Last Crossing.* Yes, that's it—a very interesting book. I am about halfway through it."

I looked quizzically at the husband, who nodded in agreement, so I continued the interview with questions about some current events and newspaper reports, which she accounted for quite accurately.

"I use these questions at least as much as the formal mental status examination to give me an idea of real, meaningful function," I explained to the resident. We agreed to continue the treatment, and, over the next two years, until she started deteriorating again, our book discussions continued as a means of monitoring her progress. In fact, she would often bring me a book to read that she had enjoyed herself.

*   *   *

Some of the more dramatic cases that taught me a lot about the elderly occurred in the acute hospital setting where I continued to see patients, most often consulting to see if I could arrange their transfer to Baycrest. (It took a long time before my colleagues gradually accepted that, in my clinical role, I might actually offer more than assisting them to empty one of their precious beds.) Many of the unusual cases occurred in patients whom I saw on behalf of surgeons who were facing an increasing number of elderly patients hoping to benefit from new technologies of surgery. One such case occurred as the techniques for correction of blindness associated with long-standing diabetes were enhanced. One of my colleagues from medical residency days was a pioneer in this field. I had not seen him for many years as our paths of travel had taken very different directions. Imagine my surprise, then, when one day at Mt. Sinai Hospital in Toronto, the elevator door opened, I entered, and there, facing me, was David Margolis. We shared a warm and somewhat emotional greeting, for we had worked closely together as residents, just as he was deciding to focus his direction on ophthalmology.

After some discussions and exploration of our mutual areas of interest, we came to a few important decisions. First, David agreed to become one of our ophthalmology consultants at Baycrest. This meant another first-class person would come up there instead of us having to send our patients downtown. Of perhaps greater significance, he was a person who was well acquainted with Jewish values and culture and held a keen interest in geriatric ophthalmology. Secondly, he had an interest in retinal disease related to diabetes mellitus, a condition that was common in young, as well as older, people. I agreed that, as much as possible, I would handle his diabetic patients before and after their surgery—some of which would be state-of-the-art vitrectomies. This was a new procedure carried out under an operating microscope whereby small blood vessels and scar tissue that, as a consequence of long-standing diabetes, grow into the center of the eyeball and block the light from traversing it, are cut away with very fine instruments. Thirdly, I would also see all of his older patients who were admitted for any kind of surgery so that their pre- and postoperative care would be optimal and we might avoid postoperative complications.

Some months after we started working together, we fell into a nice routine. We became used to each other's rhythm of practice, and we organized a schedule and method for me to come into hospital to see his patients prior to their surgery and follow up with orders and visits after surgery. David called one afternoon and told me he had a special case that required something beyond the usual. A patient from Israel had been referred to him by a former ophthalmology post- graduate fellow who had trained with David. The patient was a man with long-standing diabetes who was blind and needed a vitrectomy. The referring physician, who now held a senior position in a hospital in Israel, said there was no one in that country able to perform the procedure, and the health insurance fund had denied insurance coverage for it to be done overseas, despite his referral.

The man, who had not been able to see anything other than light for two years, was willing to take the chance on the flight to Toronto and fund the cost of the surgery himself. He spoke only Hebrew, Yiddish, and Polish—none of which David spoke, other than the Hebrew he had learned as a youngster preparing for his Bar Mitzvah and what he used for synagogue and holiday prayers.

"Can you see him for his diabetes and take care of that, but also come into the operating room and speak to him in Hebrew during the surgery?" he asked. "I will be doing the procedure using a neuroleptic anesthetic so that he will be sufficiently awake to follow some instructions during the procedure."

I agreed and saw the patient on a Wednesday afternoon,

conducting the entire evaluation in Hebrew, which, surprisingly, was still pretty good almost three years after coming to Canada after having lived in Israel for four years. The patient was shocked and delighted that he could speak to a doctor directly in his own language. Though his daughter, who had come with him, could speak some English, they both recognized the problems that are sometimes associated with translating important issues of health. Early on Thursday morning, I made a special trip downtown for the surgery and gowned up for the operating room. Everything was set up, and David had arranged for a second set of viewfinders so I could see what was going on in the eye as he operated—just one eye, on this occasion, to see if the surgery could be successful. Chaim, the patient, came in having had some preoperative sedation, but was awake. He recognized my name and voice.

"Chaim, *boker tov* (good morning)," I said in Hebrew. "I will be speaking to you during the surgery, and you will need to help us by listening carefully and following my instructions. If you have a problem, let me know so that Dr. Margolis can take the necessary steps to make the surgery a success—okay?"

"Okay," he replied.

I wished him all the best as David began to get things ready for the surgery, and the anesthetist positioned himself to administer the anesthetic, which had to be carefully controlled to achieve its goal without putting the patient out so he could respond to instructions or express problems.

Watching the probes and instruments through the operating microscope was a fantasy in real time. Gradually, I could see dense scar tissue being removed and the retina coming into focus. In the back of the eye were many areas with small hemorrhages, but the main problem was the growth of scar tissue, which was disappearing with David's expert use of the microscopic knife. "Are you okay?" I asked Chaim from time to time, asking him to squeeze my hand if "yes" and to stroke it if "no." Things were going well.

"Stop!" Chaim indicated with two strokes of my hand. Then he spoke, "I need to take a deep breath and do not want to move in a way that might upset things." David told me to tell him that it was fine for him to do so. Chaim took a few deep breaths, got back into his rhythm, and indicated that David could start again. Two hours later, David said we were done. Chaim's eye was treated with some drops and covered. We left the operating room.

"Whew!" David exclaimed. "That was a long one. There was a lot of tissue to remove, but the retina looked not bad. If he doesn't have any bleeding, I think it could be pretty good. We'll know by Saturday. I'll have a look tomorrow to make sure things seem okay, and then, on Saturday, we can have a proper look."

"I will check his sugars all day tomorrow, but will not be in the hospital—unless something happens—and then, of course, I will come down," I added.

It was Saturday morning—*Shabbat*. Neither David, the patient, nor I was particularly observant but, in any event, in situations where serious illness and health were involved, breaking the Sabbath would be permitted. However, this was not an issue among those looking after Chaim. The team stood around: David, the charge nurse, two ophthalmology residents, the patient's daughter Carmela, and me. David peeled off the bandage covering the eye. He looked at the eye and asked, "Chaim—can you see?" Turning to me, he asked me to say it in Hebrew.

But, before I could ask him, Chaim blurted out in Hebrew, "I can see, I can see! I can see you, Doctor David! I can see you, Doctor Michael. I can see!" He asked Carmela if she would call home so he could tell his wife, Simcha, the good news. It took a while for us to get a connection to Israel. We could hear the phone ringing, even though the receiver was held to Chaim's ear. "*Allo*" we heard on the other end, as a woman's voice spoke through the phone.

"Simcha," he said in Hebrew, and continued, "I can see, yes I can see. Do you understand? I can see!"

Carmela was crying, the nurses were crying, and David was smiling, also holding back tears. I could hear Simcha's voice on the other end.

"Really, Chaim, is it true?"

I asked if I could speak on the phone for a minute. I introduced myself and said to Simcha, "Dr. Margolis performed the surgery the day before yesterday, and everything seems to be okay. He can see. We will watch him carefully, but so far everything is proceeding just as we hoped it would."

"Thank God, thank God!" she kept saying. "Please give me back to Chaim."

They spoke some more and hung up. The team left, after explaining the recovery process to Chaim and Carmela, and told him when he might go home. Chaim took a wad of American dollars out of a pouch that he was wearing around his neck. "Let me pay you, please."

David said, "Chaim, this will be dealt with by the hospital, not me. Don't worry; we will make sure you can go home and everything will be taken care of." We went to the nursing station where David wrote his notes, and I followed up with mine, writing some orders for Chaim's insulin.

David turned to me and asked, "Now how about that for drama?" And we both started to laugh … just enough to hold back our tears.

*   *   *

Some time later, Dr. Margolis and I collaborated on another case, in which a frail elder was able to benefit from a cataract extraction under circumstances that had not been initially considered positive for the procedure. David asked me about a resident in the Baycrest Home for the Aged who had a reputation for being a "screamer" (someone who spent a good deal of time yelling out). It was never clear to the nurses or to his family what he was yelling about. Sometimes it had been attributed perhaps to physical discomfort, but a real cause could not be found, and simple analgesia (various mild pain medications) did not seem to have a beneficial effect.

On a routine eye examination, he was found to have dense cataracts on both eyes. Initially, the family was reluctant to consider the surgery, as their father had some degree of dementia and they were worried about possible deleterious effects. After David explained that the surgery could be carried out under local anesthetic, and I could find no medical reason to reject the possibility, we had another meeting with the family. They finally agreed that, for purposes of quality of life, he should undergo the procedure. It went well—without a hitch—and, like magic, within a few days of the patch coming off his eye, he had stopped yelling and had begun to interact meaningfully with those around him. He was, of course, still cognitively impaired, but he was no longer visually disconnected from the world. He loved to sit by the elevators, watch the people getting on and off, and kibitz with them, though in his own limited way. Now, all his screaming made sense. He had simply been crying for connection.

*   *   *

During the past few years, the medical profession and the lay public have become more aware of the potential side effects of some of the mood- and behavior-altering drugs that we often use in older people—often those with dementia— who become agitated and cannot be managed by healthcare staff or by their own families. Years ago, we were not as aware of the problems with these drugs, but, at times, it became apparent that their use was associated with many symptoms that were otherwise attributed to age and dementia.

I was asked to see an eighty-year-old man who was referred

to the clinic by his physician at the request of the patient's children. For the past two years, he had been at home and deteriorating gradually in his mental and physical function. He was less and less able to walk without assistance, and required help in some of the ordinary activities of daily living such as going to the toilet, getting dressed, and taking a shower. The family said that he had just "slowed up," more so recently, but that it had started after he had been hospitalized the year before with a severe infection. As they were telling me the story, I was taking notes and looking over his medications. He was being prescribed Haloperidol in a fairly large dose. They said he had left the hospital with it and was told it was necessary to treat his agitation and behavioral abnormalities, which the treating doctor attributed to Alzheimer's disease. As I continued to hear the story, I began looking more intently at the patient and saw that he was fairly immobile and that his face was quite expressionless.

"We wondered how he got Alzheimer's so fast," said one of his daughters, "because—before the infection—although he was occasionally forgetful, he was still living on his own and was not having many problems. After he left the hospital, we had to get help for him, and things really never got better. If anything, he is less mobile now and less communicative than he was two years ago." The examination revealed severe abnormalities in his movements—the kind that one often sees with Parkinson's disease. I reviewed all of his other medications, and none of them could be implicated in what appeared to be severe side effects of the Haloperidol. Moreover, the history, and a copy of the discharge summary from that hospitalization sent along by the referring physician, confirmed the family's comments that prior to that hospitalization he had been functioning reasonably well. The hospitalization appeared to have been precipitated by a severe urinary tract infection, which had been treated; then, a prostate problem, which seemed to be the cause of the urinary infection, was also corrected. But, because he had become very agitated and combative during the infection and, again, after the surgery, he was put on the Haloperidol and discharged home with it, without any instructions to discontinue it once he got better.

Because he was so slow, it was impossible to tell from the examination what the status of his mental or cognitive function might be. I assumed that it might be impaired, but that his Parkinson-like symptoms were probably due to the drug. I instructed the daughters in how to incrementally taper the drug off over the following three weeks and asked them to bring him back to the office in six weeks' time. When he arrived at that visit, he was a different person. He walked in unaided and, not only could smile at me, but he spoke in sentences. There was evidence of some mild cognitive impairment, but, according to the daughters, his general function was not all that different from how he had been the year before prior to his hospitalization. The patient and his daughters were most pleased—as I was, too—to have such a simple intervention result in so dramatic an improvement. As they left, one of the daughters leaned over to me and said, "Thank you for giving our father back to us."

Powerful drugs that affect the brain are often prescribed in situations for which they are not really required, or they are needed only on a temporary basis, but are not discontinued. As a result, adverse drug reactions are common in the elderly, and this overmedication is a condition for which those of us who work in the field of geriatrics must remain ever vigilant.

*　　　*　　　*

"So where are you from? Tell me about yourself—not your illness yet … just about you. That sounds like a Scottish accent—are you a Scot?"

"How do you know?" he answered with a broad smile.

I often start my medical interviews with a question that

tries to probe the identity of the person I will be treating, as a means of finding a way to make a personal connection. Over the years, I have had many wonderful experiences and have shared many wonderful stories with patients because of such opening questions, and I have always taught my residents that making that connection can have an impact on the future of a doctor-patient relationship.

"It's hard to miss with your accent, and I bet you're from Dundee."

His wife, sitting next to him aside his daughter, said in an accent from the north of England, "I hope you can understand him; I've lived with him for fifty years and I still can't." We conversed in the broadest Dundee I could muster after so many years, managing to hit some of the highlights of the city that he had left in the 1950s but that, clearly, had not changed that much by the '60s when I lived there.

"De ya ken (Do you know) the Deep Sea Fish shop on the Perth Road?" I asked.

"Aye, fine place, gid fud (good food)," he answered. We went back and forth for a few more sentences when his daughter, a woman in her forties, added, "I always struggled to understand my father; he and mother seemed to be speaking different languages all the time—I guess it really is a different language." We all shared a good laugh and went on to medicine.

*   *   *

"That's a fairly well-known name," I said. "Are you related to the famous judge and the professor of medicine?" I asked the sprightly lady who came to the office on her own, in itself an uncommon event since almost everyone came with a family member.

"Yes, they are two of my sons. Do you know them?"

"I know the doctor because we have met at medical

conferences, and the judge only by reputation. But, if that is the case, your granddaughter must be Anna."

She looked at me with wide eyes. "How do you know the name of my granddaughter? Do you know her?"

"She shares an apartment with my daughter Neta. They were in high school together."

"Your daughter is Neta? I know Neta. She has been to my home with Anna. She is a lovely girl."

From then on, this patient was like a family member, and every visit would begin with a rundown of her family, with a special focus on her beloved granddaughter. About a year later, I met her physician son at a medical conference, and he related back to me how much his mother enjoyed the medical visits and how fond she was of me.

*   *   *

I was trying to explain to my medical resident the meaning of a Yiddish word that I was using when speaking with a Jewish woman who was clearly of Eastern European origins and whose mother tongue, I figured, was Yiddish.

"Mrs. Eckstein, I am not going to make a *tsimmis* of my going over the story again with you that the young doctor just spent an hour doing—just so I can hear some of the points directly."

"A *tsimmis* should be a carrot *tsimmis*," she said. "I am a *Litvak*."

I explained to the resident that a *Litvak* was someone from Lithuania and that a *tsimmis* was a special holiday stew that had different contents depending on the Eastern European country of origin. "Mrs. Eckstein, my grandparents were *Litvaks* as well, so I know what a carrot *tsimmis* is. My grandmother, who lived with me in Brooklyn, used to make it. She came from Eyshoshuk."

The patient almost bolted from her chair, "Eyshoshuk!

That is where I am from. I left in 1939 just after the invasion of Poland, and we went east to Siberia. I can't believe this. What was their name?"

"Gordon and Levine," I told her.

"I am sure my parents knew them. I can't believe this; we are landsmen." I explained to the resident that this meant someone from the same village. We talked about the history of the town and the famous book written about it—*There Once Was a World*—and how there were no Jews left in that village as they had all been murdered during the war. It was a profound experience and, for the patient, a connection to her history and to me, as her doctor.

*   *   *

Sometimes physicians do their best to convince patients of the necessity of a treatment, and, no matter how hard the physician tries or how compelling the physician believes the logic might be behind the treatment, the patient refuses. This can even occur when the treatment is very likely to be beneficial—even lifesaving—and when, unlike with some other treatments, the risk of having the procedure is very small.

"I will not have any heart surgery," was the adamant reply from Samuel Wolfson, an eighty-two-year-old man living in a retirement residence where I ran a geriatric clinic every week. "I am too old and will not have anybody cutting me open."

I tried to explain. "Mr. Wolfson, this is not surgery the way you think of a really big operation. It is hardly surgery at all. Putting in a pacemaker has become a very minor procedure, and the cut is just a small incision to put in the pacemaker unit, which is much smaller than a hockey puck." Samuel had been having fainting spells out of the blue, and a twenty-four-hour continuous Holter monitor had revealed, without question, pauses in his heart conduction that required a pacemaker to prevent a stoppage that could be lethal—either because the heart might not start again or, more likely, because the stoppage could lead to a serious fall and a fracture or injury to his head.

I was running out of arguments. I had even tried bringing in Eva, another resident of the retirement home who, the year before, successfully had had a pacemaker inserted and no longer suffered from falls. (A previous one had resulted in a broken arm; she had been lucky.) Eva agreed to speak to Samuel, whom she knew from some of the social programs they attended together. She would speak to him about what a simple procedure it was and how much it had helped her.

"Samuel, don't be foolish. This is not a heart operation. It is over in an hour or two. I was home the evening of the day they did it. You hardly know you have the thing in place—it is just under the skin." She was a very open and dramatic speaker. At this point, to his surprise, she grabbed his hand and pulled it up to just above her left breast and said, "Here, feel it? You would hardly know it's there. It's not very big, you see. Can you feel anything?"

I could see the look of slight embarrassment on his face as she pushed his hand to just above her left breast and pushed it around. The pacemaker would have been just underneath his hand. After she left, he said, "I don't think so. Thank you for trying to convince me. I think I will just let whatever happens, happen."

I could not think of anything else to say. But then I thought for a moment and asked, "Samuel, what kind of work did you do before you retired?" I knew from his accent that he was probably an Eastern European immigrant, but his English was very good and very fluent, with only the mildest hint of an accent. He looked at me and said, "I was a traveling salesman—ladies' garments. I represented some of the best manufacturers in Toronto and drove all over the country. In those days, it was the only way. The car was full of samples, and I just drove from town to town and visited all the shops. Some were already established customers, and some were potential customers. I did it for thirty years, and only retired when the driving became too much for me."

"You must have either loved the driving or had a lot of patience," I added.

"I actually loved the driving. I tried to keep it to two- or three-week trips at the most, with a good break in between. I was away a lot from home. My family understood, and I made a good living—hard work, yes, but it kept us going with a pretty nice lifestyle and sent my children for their education. It was pretty good."

"Samuel," I pursued, "I was wondering, with all that driving, what kind of car did you drive? You must have needed something reliable."

"I owned and drove only Oldsmobiles—the '88 model with the V8 engine. What a car ... it never let me down. I kept them in good shape, mind you—oil changes, brakes, and good tires ... what a car."

"So, I guess when the battery went dead, you just dumped the car—got rid of it?"

Samuel looked at me incredulously. "Why would anyone dump an '88 because of a bum battery? No, I would get a new battery."

"Did that ever happen to any of your cars?" I asked conversationally.

"Of course! Once—in Winnipeg, I remember—it got real cold, and I guess I had kept the battery a bit too long. I was supposed to drive to Brandon, but the car was dead. It took a few hours, but, with a new battery, I was on my way—that car could really drive. And, even with the delay, I got there just a bit later than I had planned."

"Samuel, that's exactly what I have been trying to tell you. You are better than an '88! You are a great model person, but your battery is not working—in fact, it is a bum battery that may soon give out. What you need is a new battery—that is what a pacemaker is ... a new battery for a great model. Don't throw the model away—it's got lots of miles left in it."

Samuel looked at me. Clearly, I had given it my last best shot. He broke into a smile. "Now that you explain it that way, I understand. Sure, I will get a new battery—what do I have to do? And naturally, doctor, I want the best brand you can get," he said with a broad grin.

We shook hands and I told him we would make the arrangements.

*   *   *

Sometimes events occur in my office that might be considered outside the normal expectations or activities involved in a visit to the doctor. Some of these events are memorable and add to the abundance that forms the menu of geriatric practice. On one particular day, it happened that two of my long-standing patients—unrelated to one another and at different times of the day—sang for me as part of their visits. Why might a patient sing for the doctor? While it could be that I was a medical specialist who focused on singers with voice problems, that is, clearly, not the case. As a geriatrician, the majority of my patients are in their eighties and nineties and are no longer employed.

The first patient was a renowned cantor who was afflicted with Parkinson's disease. Along with his family and treating physicians, he struggled to find ways to improve his function. At one point, he could not vocalize sufficiently to sing. Fortunately, there was some return of function as we altered medications and juggled the doses so that, during the best of times, he was once again able to sing a short, beautiful, and sustained cantorial tune. On this particular day, after we had chatted for a while, out it suddenly came—a beautiful and lyrical sound—first in the office and, then, as he demonstrated his gait in the hallway, so that everyone in the vicinity could benefit from the purity of his sound. He smiled with pleasure as passersby stopped to listen to the long, drawn-out notes.

The second patient was a woman who was always accompanied by one, if not two, very devoted family members. She suffered from dementia, but still lived with her family, who were very supportive of maintaining her at home rather than moving her into a nursing home. Ever since I met her, she had told me how much she loved to sing. Some years ago during the early part of our interaction, I told her that my maternal grandmother, who helped raise me in Brooklyn, sang in the Yiddish choir in New York. I told her that I had heard lots of Yiddish singing as a child, and had accompanied my grandmother on the piano when she practiced for performances. Invariably, after our medical visit, the patient would tell me she was going to sing me a Yiddish song. In the earlier days, she would sing one of a number of songs with all the lyrics intact. As time went by and her language skills deteriorated with the progress of dementia, the lyrics became less robust, but the melody remained true, her voice clear and sweet sounding. The recent visit ended with her singing My Yiddish Mamma, in which the only words were those in the title—and the rest was humming and la- la- la-ing—but on beat and in tune. I sat, smiling at her as she sang, and, when she was finished, I told her how much I enjoyed her singing for me. When I asked if she would come to see me again for a follow-up appointment, she smiled and said, "Of course, doctor; I always like to come and sing for you."

Over the years, many of my medical colleagues have questioned how I am able to look after patients who are old, have many illnesses, and may be quite demented. "How can you speak to them with any real satisfaction?" I am often asked. I have frequently heard from medical trainees that some of their supervisors paint a rather negative picture of eldercare. I am saddened by this, as many of these young medical students and postgraduate trainees have a natural inclination toward the elderly. While I try to counter the negativity of others, sometimes I do not succeed in doing so. Working in a clinic in which two patients sing to me on the same day is the perfect and lyrical antidote.

*   *   *

Sometimes a patient's illness may only become apparent after some critical event or after another physician sees the patient with "new eyes." I often teach my residents that the reason consultations are often helpful is not just that the person you are referring to has special or unique knowledge—which, of course, is usually the case—but that a consulting physician is looking at the patient with new eyes and listening with new ears. One such case was remarkable in that the patient had a condition with a severity that I had not seen since medical school.

At the time I saw her, she was in her later seventies. Her younger sister worked as a volunteer in the outpatient clinic area where my geriatric clinic was situated. Through the family doctor, the sister had arranged for me to see her older sibling because the sister was always tired. "I know you can be tired when you get close to eighty years old," she told me, "but this is just not like her—all she wants to do is sleep. She has also gained quite a lot of weight." A few weeks later, the older sister walked into my office, and, as soon as she entered the examining room, I said to the resident who was with me, "What does she have?"

The resident looked at her and said, "I need to take a history—I am not sure."

I greeted the patient, who replied with a rough raspy voice, "What's the diagnosis?" I asked again. The resident asked if she could ask some questions. She ascertained that the patient was tired, always sleeping, and had gained a lot of weight. I then asked again, "Think—weight gain, fatigue, and—look at her face." It was the height of summer. I asked the patient, "When you are at home these days, do you feel you need to wear a sweater?" The patient answered, "I am always cold; no matter what, I am always cold. I am always turning the air conditioner off, and I walk around in a sweater."

By this time, the resident had put the puzzle together. "She is hypothyroid. But how did you know before you asked her some questions?"

I explained, "When I was in medical school, we had a patient with similar symptoms, and the chief of medicine did pretty much what I have done here with you. When I asked how he knew the diagnosis, he said, 'She looks just like Aunt Mary!'" He went on to explain that he had an aunt who developed not just hypothyroidism, but a very severe case of myxedema, in which the characteristic look included a bloated, heavy, pasty appearance to the face, and a deep hoarse voice. So the typical appearance led to the diagnosis even without taking a real history. Of course, with the history, the story fit even more into place—with the cold intolerance and weight gain. And, when the resident examined her, she found the other characteristic features, such as dry skin. What was interesting is that the patient had had a pacemaker put in not long before for a very slow heart rate, and I wondered if the doctor had considered the possibility of low thyroid levels when he did it.

We started the patient on the correct replacement thyroid hormone, and sent a letter to the family doctor, with a copy to the cardiologist. Over the next few months, she improved dramatically, with her face returning to its previous thin appearance (the sister had brought in a picture that was a few years old so that I could evaluate the changes). Her voice improved, as did her skin texture, but, most importantly, the perpetual fatigue disappeared. A few weeks after I had seen her in this much improved condition and wrote a follow-up letter to both physicians, I received a phone call from the cardiologist admitting to me that he had missed the thyroid diagnosis altogether. To his credit, it sounded as if the condition had not been as obvious as it was when I saw her, but he felt that her very slow heart rate had very likely been due to her thyroid, and he had not considered the possibility before he inserted the pacemaker. With treatment, her heart rate returned to normal, and the cardiogram showed that the pacemaker no longer activated because the heart's speed was no longer slow.

*   *   *

Should our medical careers span long periods of time, most of us will become aware of conditions that may not have been recognized previously, or may not have been well described. Some may write up case reports or describe groups of patients with conditions that appear to be new, different, or a variation of a previously known condition, and add these observations to the medical literature. Within a few years of my beginning this specialized geriatric practice, I had seen a variety of patients who complained that, when they walked, they became exceedingly tired and sometimes a bit short of breath, and, when they stopped walking, the symptoms would resolve. Then they would carry on again for a while, and then the cycle would start all over again. Some of these patients had known heart disease, and some did not. What was peculiar was that a number of these patients did not complain of chest pain, pressure, or any other symptom when they were having these attacks that might have suggested the clinical condition of angina.

Wondering if they might have an underlying lung problem, I sent a few for further investigation, but the tests all turned out normal. This was a time when Holter monitors for the heart were relatively accurate at measuring the rhythm, but not much else, so the technology could not be used to see changes in the appearance of the heart's electrical impulse that might be found with poor blood flow (ischemia) to the heart muscle. For a reason that was not so clear-cut in my thinking, I suggested that one of these patients try taking a nitroglycerin tablet under his tongue (as he would for angina with its typical associated chest pain) before he went for the kind of walk in which he would get short of breath or tired. We would then see if it made a difference.

I saw him a few weeks later. "It was magic!" he said with glee. "No shortness of breath. I could walk! I can't believe it." At that point, I gave him a long-acting nitrate instead of the nitroglycerin under the tongue. He took this a few times a day, and, at a later visit, told me that now he hardly had any episodes at all. A few weeks later, I had a similar case in which the same symptoms occurred. At a journal club meeting of our geriatric group, I humorously postulated that I was seeing cases of "painless angina." After a few guffaws from my colleagues, I explained that what I thought was happening was the typical angina event in people who did not experience the episode as the usual pain but, instead, felt fatigue or shortness of breath—what I suggested were angina equivalents that were not painful. They listened and said they would look for such patients as well. I saw a few more and mentioned it to a cardiology friend who thought I might be right, though he could not recall seeing such a patient. He admitted that his practice did not have many extremely elderly patients, and most came to him for advice on treatment with already diagnosed heart disease. I gradually accumulated a few more cases and became convinced that painless angina was a real entity, and even wrote an editorial about it suggesting the use of anti-angina therapy in such cases as a therapeutic trial.

The editorial was initially rejected, but, on appeal to the editor with some supporting data, it was accepted and published in 1986 with a counter editorial by a cardiologist.

About a year later, I was at a geriatric conference overseas and attended a presentation by a nuclear medicine expert on new findings using cardiac scanning. Interestingly, this technology demonstrated changes of ischemia in patients who did not complain of pain—in fact, he used the word "silent ischemia." I spoke to him afterward and related my experiences to him and my use of the term "silent angina," to which he replied, "That's what it is!" I felt vindicated, and now had the kind of scientific evidence a physician always needs to support clinical observations, especially when they are new or appear to be in conflict with established knowledge. This anecdote is also an example of the kind of tension and excitement that exists within medical practice and why, even in the world of modern medicine, the individual doctor remains at the core of medical observation and serves as the basis for all future medical progress.

*　　　*　　　*

Much has been written in the past few years about the stigma associated with mental health conditions and how, in general, physicians and the public ignore or shun individuals with mental health problems, especially depression. Even with the advent of potent medications and other effective therapies for depression, it has been common—even until the present time—for older individuals with depression to have their symptoms missed or confused with other conditions that affect the elderly. The most common and, until a few years ago, worst possible misreading of the symptoms of late-age depression was the assumption that the forgetfulness and lack of interest characteristic of depression was simply the manifestation of dementia. In earlier days before the development of effective, symptomatic treatment for dementia, a misinterpretation of the symptoms was even more significant, for antidepressants might not be prescribed and that would be the end of the story.

A grandson, now a surgeon and one of my interns some years before, said of his grandmother, "She is just not the same. She is not speaking as much, seems to want to be just left alone, and, most important, has given up bridge. My mother, who sees her most, says she simply will not go to the games any more. She claims that she cannot concentrate and is 'no use' to her partner."

I spoke to the eighty-three-year-old woman while, with her permission, the grandson remained with us in the room. As he had said, it seemed that she just did not seem to be that interested in anything, and admitted, "I think it's time. I have had a good life. What else is there? I can't even enjoy bridge anymore, and that was really my favorite activity."

The grandson recounted that his grandmother had been quite a bridge player and had still been participating in tournaments until this change came about.

"I think you are depressed and not suffering from a dementia like Alzheimer's disease," I told her.

"Why would I be depressed? I have wonderful children and grandchildren—look at him … already a surgeon—I am very proud of him."

I explained that depression, like many other illnesses, does not always have an obvious cause, and having a good life was no protection from it.

"Well, I am not sure," she said. "I don't think I will be playing bridge again."

I discussed treatment with antidepressant medications. I had been using one at the time that also had a fairly good sedative effect—she was also complaining of problems with her sleeping. "I get up at night, sometimes at three in the morning, and cannot go back to sleep. I just lie there, thinking of my past and all the things I wish I had done differently."

She agreed to try the medications. Two weeks later, the grandson called to bring me up-to-date, saying, "I think she is improving—for sure her sleep is better—and she seems somewhat less withdrawn." I asked him to tell her to increase the dosage, as I had started with a very low dose to avoid any possible side effects. Six weeks later, she came into my office looking completely different.

"I played bridge this past weekend. I was not great, but I managed. My sleep is pretty good as well."

I modified the dose a bit more, and, three months later, the grandson called to report, "She is back to her old self—playing bridge and socializing."

From her case and many others, over the years I have come to appreciate the power of depression and its terrible impact on older people. That there is hope must be emphasized to them. There are therapies, including medications that can be tried so that eventually, even when there are difficulties sometimes, treatment is often successful.

I often meet people—including other physicians—who, when I mention that I am a geriatrician, either grimace at the thought or commend me for "doing something so important" even though masked behind their comments is often the thought of "I wonder how anyone would pick that line of work?" or "How depressing it must be to take care of people at the end of their lives, who often are impaired and dependent on others." The reality is quite the opposite. From a medical point of view, caring for older people is always clinically and intellectually challenging. But, more than that, the practice brings to the physician and other healthcare professionals involved a sense of personal history, humor, grief, joy, and the rich experiences that have been part of the older person's life. I have always marveled at the power of the experience of providing care to this wonderful generation of elders who have experienced many of the great global events that have affected my personal history. More importantly, their personal experiences and stories have taught me much, and my life has been enriched through an association with each one.

Chapter 11

Sojourn in the Arab World

"I'm from Palestine, from Nablus," said the young reporter who was interviewing me at a conference on aging in Doha, Qatar. "Do you know where that is?"

"Of course I know where Nablus is!" I replied. "I lived in Israel for four years in the early seventies. I worked in Ramallah helping to set up the region's first nursing school."

The reporter looked at me, and then asked me in Hebrew, "So you speak Hebrew?" to which I replied, also in Hebrew, "Of course. How is it that you speak it?"

"I worked as an Arabic-Hebrew translator. But I haven't had the chance to speak it in the more than eight months that I have been living here," he replied.

Yet here we were, in a busy pressroom in the Doha Ritz-Carlton surrounded by reporters from all the Middle Eastern and Gulf Arab press, carrying out an interview for the *Gulf Times*, the regional English-language daily, entirely in Hebrew. No one seemed to be the least bit interested or concerned. When the interview was over, we said our good-byes in English, and then I added in my most basic Arabic, "*Salem Aleykum.*"

He smiled and returned the similar Hebrew greeting, "*Shalom Aleichem.*"

I had been invited to two back-to-back conferences hosted by the government of Qatar on behalf of the Gulf and Middle Eastern Arabic countries, to share information and knowledge on primary care and the care of the elderly. The region is developing rapidly and thus beginning to experience an aging population. My host was a physician from Qatar who had spent two years in Toronto, one of these at Baycrest studying family medicine and the care of the elderly. He had a particular interest in medical ethics, and had attended many of the seminars on the subject that I had led. I was invited to speak at these conferences because of my professional experience in geriatrics, but also my special interest in ethics and *Halacha* (Jewish Law). I had been asked to incorporate my knowledge of other religions into the discussion. Being Jewish, and never having traveled to a modern-day Arabic nation—other than a one-day excursion trip from Eilat in Israel to Petra in Jordan—I was a little unsure of what to expect. I did not really consider as a visit the brief time I spent in Tunisia in 1967 to visit my sister in the Peace Corps where I ended up experiencing the Six-Day War through Arab media. Rather, that had been a life-changing experience.

Years before, though, I had had some meaningful experiences engaging with the Arab world. I had worked in three Israeli hospitals—one in Haifa and two in Jerusalem—for several years: in 1965 as a medical student, in 1967 as an intern, and then from 1971 to 1973 as a medical resident. This period of my medical training introduced me to the Arab culture, since Arabs made up a large proportion of the patient population in each of the hospitals where I had worked. Israeli hospitals were open to everyone, and many of the most complex patients were Arabs who came from all over the country for care, often preferring the Israeli hospitals over their local hospitals or the ethnically focused hospital for

Arabs which existed in Jerusalem. I had treated many Arab patients over the years; some very challenging cases had come into Shaare Zedek Hospital where I completed two years of medical residency, a position that included running the intensive care unit for six months.

One of the most dramatic cases we dealt with during that time was a farmer from a small West Bank Arab village, brought in by his family because he was having "fits." After an initial assessment in the emergency room, it became clear that he, in fact, had tetanus, which I had never seen before. Only one of the staff physicians had ever treated a case, and that had been many years previously, and the outcome had been unsuccessful.

During these fits, the patient experienced contractions every few minutes, lasting up to a minute, during which time his back was arched and he was very stiff, his breathing was strained, and his eyes rolled back. It seemed that almost anything—noise or even touch—would set him off. We had one of our Abu Gosh Israeli-Arab university students who assisted us on the units translate to the family and tell them on our behalf just how ill he was. After searching carefully, we found what we thought was likely the infective source: a cut on his foot. Such cuts and abrasions of the feet were common in farmers. Since this was long before the development of an accessible electronic repository of information, we manually searched the library for sources that would describe treatments, but many were out-of-date. We felt the most likely other treatment—besides the anti-tetanus toxin we had administered in the emergency room—was to put him on an infusion of the tranquilizer Valium. We could only guess at the dose, just as we would have done in a patient with uncontrolled epileptic seizures. After the initial dose, we would titrate the Valium; in other words, try to determine the amount he needed based on its apparent effect on his condition. He was moved to the intensive care unit, now under my direction as the senior resident, and members of the family were allowed in two at a time for brief visits. They hovered and watched intently over the first few hours as the frequency and intensity of the contractions decreased.

Our translator told them to go home and come back in the morning, for his condition was serious and this was going to be a long treatment process. As they left, they blessed each of the staff—doctors and nurses—and we, in turn, wished them well. Even though I was not on duty that night, I stayed in the hospital. The house officer on call was rather junior, and I could see he felt a bit insecure about titrating the Valium infusion, since too much of the drug could lethally halt the patient's respirations. By the morning, we had reasonably controlled the seizures. The challenge was the nursing care of the patient: we were worried that he might develop pressure ulcers, but each necessary position movement to fight this could trigger a serious contraction. The nurses started to develop inventive techniques for the changes and movements; for example, with some extra doses of drug prior to the move, we managed to limit the number and intensity of the attacks.

Ensuring adequate nutrition was also a concern as we realized that intravenous fluids alone would not sustain him for very long. We decided to insert a nasogastric feeding tube—a pediatric one for comfort—using a trick I had learned some years before as, normally, a thin pediatric plastic tube curls up at the back of the mouth as it is being inserted through the nose of an adult. Here's the trick: we attached the pediatric tube side by side to a regular-size plastic feeding tube and held the two of them together at the end with half a tetracycline (an antibiotic) capsule, knowing that it would dissolve when it entered the stomach. We put the two tubes into ice so that they became stiff, then put on lots of lubricant. Then, with a careful synchronization with his breathing to make sure we did not insert it while he was inhaling, we successfully slipped in the tubes. After a few moments, we flushed some saline first down the large tube and then down the small tube, and then we pulled the large tube out, checking to be sure that the pediatric tube was in place. It worked! We now had a method for sustaining his nutrition over the period that we hoped was necessary for the tetanus toxin to dissipate and his contractions to stop. Over the following week, we tried to wean him off the Valium, but his contractions recurred, so we waited. Finally, after ten days, we were able to carry out the weaning over two days until, finally, he was not receiving any Valium. He opened his eyes and saw his family sitting around him, said a few words, and there were hugs and kisses all round. One of the older members of the family came over to me, bowed, and took my hand and kissed it. A week later, the farmer went home—a bit gaunt, but without any pressure ulcers and, against all of our expectations, and his family's, alive.

*   *   *

The drama of this tetanus case reminds me of my first experience with an Arab family. It occurred on my first visit to Israel, when I was a medical student working in the Rambam Hospital in Haifa. A large Israeli-Arab community was served by Rambam Hospital, and families would often be seen sitting on the lawn outside the hospital, sometimes joined by what was clearly an ill relative who, while still needing to be hospitalized, was well enough to leave the ward for a while. The staff on the unit knew that I was very keen to do anything exciting. Criteria for participation as a medical student at the hospital would be considered rather loose by today's standards. My training in Scotland was deemed good enough to permit me to do anything an Israeli student or intern might do, as long as language did not get in the way. The language issue was rare, as almost all the doctors spoke English, and many of the patients did as well—at least enough to allow me to practice medicine. The arrangement turned out to be mutually beneficial: I loved the exposure and excitement; the interns loved that I was willing to hang around the ward and do "scut" work (the ordinary daily activities on the ward that more senior residents often think of as routine and not very interesting like taking blood samples and putting in intravenous infusions) and "scrub in" (be an assistant at surgery)—especially on the gynecological procedures, which, for them, were routine and repetitious. The staff physicians and professor loved having me there and were happy to explain to me in English what they were doing.

One afternoon, soon after lunch when there were no staff physicians on the unit and things were on the quiet side, I heard a lot of commotion. A patient, who happened to be an Arab woman, was wheeled into the procedure room, screaming and lashing out. Her husband was frantically trying to calm her down while explaining to the nurse, who spoke some Arabic, that his wife was experiencing a great deal of pain. He knew she was pregnant, but it was much too early for her to be delivered. The nurse initially assumed it was an early labor, but, as she started examining the patient, I could see from her face that she was becoming worried. She told the other nurse to get Dr. Levy, the on-call doctor, and tell him it was urgent. In the meantime, they would get everything ready for an infusion and taking blood for a transfusion. I was the only medical person in the department at the time. The senior staff person arrived and after speaking to the husband and the patient who, by now, was not looking well at all, told the nurse to call down to the operating room to prepare for an emergency laparotomy (an incision into the abdominal wall, in this case for exploratory purposes).

"I think we have an ectopic—get some O-negative blood—and get an IV in her fast!" (An ectopic pregnancy is one in which the fertilized egg develops outside the womb (uterus), often in the Fallopian tubes, which lead from the ovaries to the uterus. Because the space is very small, there is a high risk of rupture of the Fallopian tube and severe and life-threatening bleeding.) The IV kit was brought over and given to me. I put the rubber tourniquet on her arm—her veins were flat.

"I think putting in a needle is dangerous as it can cut out and we can't afford that. Should I try this catheter?" It was an Intracath, a somewhat new technique for Israel, but one with which I had experience from my Scottish medical school training.

Dr. Levy looked at me and said, "If you know how to do it, fine. The anesthetist is waiting for us in the operating room to get started, and the blood is just coming up the elevator."

I asked the nurse to hold her arm down, and she asked the husband to speak to his wife to tell her to try not to move. She was still groaning and moaning even though she had been given something for pain. There were only two Intracaths on the tray and, after I cleaned the arm and rubbed the iodine on it, I looked to see if the vein had filled a bit so that I could easily enter it with the wide-bore needle. That was the problem with this technique: the needle was quite big because the plastic catheter ran up through it. There was a moment of silence as all eyes looked at me and the arm as I opened the packet, slid the sheath off the needle, and held it just below the crease in the patient's elbow. With a swift motion, I put the needle in, and, as soon as I saw the small thread of blood seep back into the catheter, I pushed it in, still holding the needle in place. It was a move I had learned in Scotland, mostly during my cardiology locum earlier that year. Luckily for us now, I had had the opportunity to perform the maneuver many times.

"We're in! Tape please—lots of it." The last thing I wanted was for this lifeline to come out.

"Very good, very good," Dr. Levy said, as he checked the blood type and told the nurse to hang it. "Wide open," he ordered. "We may need another line, but let us get her down to the OR as fast as we can." We wheeled her into the room, the swinging doors flying open, and quickly moved her to the table. I barely had time to get scrubbed and into my gown and mask to join the surgery, but did not want to miss it for the world. The anesthetist put the cuff on her arm, the mask on her face, and raised the O2 as high up as it could go.

"Get her prepped and I will tube her. Then I am putting another line in her so we can give her another unit of blood. Her pressure is low and her pulse is up."

Within minutes, Dr. Levy was slicing into the abdomen—there was lots of blood to be seen—then he put his hand in and announced, "Left side—ectopic!" He was handed a few clamps, which he began to put in place while the nurse and I suctioned the blood out as fast as we could.

As soon as the clamps were in place, the bleeding subsided and we could actually see what was there. Dr. Levy pointed everything out to me. "A few more minutes, and we could have lost her. She was bleeding a lot."

The anesthetist reported, "It's okay. Her blood pressure is up and she is stabilizing."

Dr. Levy started suturing and asked if I would like to stitch the abdomen—to which I nodded yes—and when the time came, under his careful eye, I carried out the stitching procedure I had learned so well in Scotland. This was certainly easier than the scalps in Dundee, but, since it would be seen by her husband, I wanted to do a really nice job.

*   *   *

As I had explained to the reporter in the newsroom in Doha, during the years when I lived in Israel from 1969–1973, some of my residency training took place at Jerusalem's Shaare Zedek Hospital. One day, as was his habit, David Meir, the director general, called out my name across the department of medicine ward, knowing that either I would hear him or someone else would and give me the message. "Michael, I have been asked something very unique and very special—and I need your help." My protective mode immediately went into high gear: he was a great boss, but one always knew that, when he had a project that required work, he had already made the decision as to who would take it on. "The Ministry of Health, Ministry of Interior, and Ministry of Education are undertaking a project to develop a nursing school on the West Bank to replace the one that was there before the Six-Day War and has now migrated to Jordan. They want to provide a nursing education to local girls so that they do not have to leave the region to study. Presently, they have to go to Jordan or Lebanon. I have been asked to help."

I looked at David and asked, "What does that have to do with me—it is a nursing school—why don't you speak to Tamar, the director of nursing?" He continued, "They want a physician as the course director, and someone whose mother tongue is English, since the courses will be taught in English. If possible, they said, maybe someone who is not a *Sabra* (native-born Israeli) so the students do not have to deal with Hebrew-accented English and the potential humiliation of being taught by a true Israeli." I could see the gleam in his eye as he continued, "And you are perfect for the job."

"Just a minute—when am I supposed to do this? I have my medical ward to look after."

"It is one afternoon a week, and I will make sure you have coverage so you will not have to worry about what happens when you are away." I did a quick calculation and knew that, between the half-hour drive there and back and probably two to three hours at the school, I would be away for a whole afternoon. I also knew that, when I was told "not to worry" because someone would cover me, it really meant that I would have to pick up the pieces when I returned.

But it seemed like a really interesting opportunity. The

following week, I drove to Ramallah, a town I had visited previously as a tourist. It was a popular place for Jerusalemites to go for an outing for some good dining and shopping, as the prices were actually lower than in the Jerusalem Jewish and Arab markets. Some people were leery of buying fruits and vegetables there because of what they deemed to be poor hygiene; and, admittedly, there was evidence that some farmers used sewage to fertilize fields, which increased the risk of gastrointestinal infections. Those who did buy their produce on a routine basis in Ramallah soaked the goods in purple potassium permanganate. It usually did the trick in terms of removing dangerous bacteria.

I arrived at the building that was to be the temporary home of the nursing school and met Noor, who was the director. Petite, very attractive, and full of energy, she offered me *botz* (literally "mud," but really Turkish coffee), and we sat down for two hours of planning. By the end of the meeting, I had agreed to run the program and the curriculum from the medical perspective. She would determine the nursing curriculum. The practical training would take place under the supervision of the staff at the Augusta Victoria Hospital in East Jerusalem. In the first year, I would teach anatomy and physiology and, if things worked out, would then teach medicine and surgery.

"I do not have any current textbooks," Noor told me. "We will be getting some, but you can use the big blackboard that I have purchased for the class, and I have lots of colored chalk." I learned that she had bought white and five other colors— and I figured that would be enough for my needs.

When I returned to the hospital that evening, I went to the library and found a book on anatomy and one on physiology, and I arranged with the librarian to keep them on permanent loan unless someone needed them. "Check with the director general—I am sure he will approve it," I said.

The following week, I stood in the class, having been plied

earlier with two cups of *botz*. This would become the tradition for the next two years: I would spend thirty minutes with Noor (and two cups of coffee) reviewing what was happening. After a five-minute break, I was geared up for a ninety-minute class. That first day, twenty-five girls entered the classroom, their eyes all modestly downcast. They quietly took their places at the combination desk and chair seating set out for them. Noor introduced me first with a few words of Arabic, and I greeted them with "*Salem Aleykum*," but then she announced, "In this class we will speak only English. Dr. Gordon will speak to you only in English—no Arabic and no Hebrew—is that clear?" I could hear them all quietly murmur "yes," and some of them moved their heads to look at neighboring classmates. Noor smiled at me and walked out the door, saying "Good luck," to me and, "Be good students," to the girls.

The girls looked to range from eighteen to twenty years of age. They all had dark hair, and most wore it tied in a single, long braid. From what I could see, their blouses and skirts were long, and none wore any makeup—all of this was quite a change from what I had seen of girls of this age in Jerusalem and other parts of Israel, other than in the religious community. We went around the room, and each girl told me her name and the village where she lived. Then I said, "I have a list of your names, but it will take me time to remember them and learn how to pronounce them. In the beginning before I learn them, would you please say your name first when you speak until I get to know you all?"

One girl raised her hand and asked, "May we write when you speak to us? We have all brought notebooks." She lifted up what in the United States would have been a grade school lined notebook. All the girls pulled them out of their bags and showed me theirs as well.

"Of course!" I replied. "Since I will be drawing lots of pictures, that would actually be a very good idea. You have a lot to learn ... new ideas and new words. The nursing director told me you do not have much in the way of books, but she is going to try and make some mimeographs of some of the things you will need." Twenty-five sets of eyes, mostly dark in color, but a few blue and green, stared back at me, all poised to learn.

I turned to the blackboard and took a piece of white chalk and wrote the words "Anatomy and Physiology" on the board in large letters and asked, "What do these words mean to you?" I was pleasantly surprised by the answers. There was some reluctance in many of the girls to answer, so I started going around the room for answers, telling them not to be afraid of giving a wrong answer, for that is how we learn. That concept seemed to surprise them. By the end of the second lesson, each of them had said something in class, and I was beginning to remember some names; Fatima, Sameeha, Mahdeyeh, Aidah, Akila, Badra, Daliyah, Fahima, Hana, Lunah, Mariam, Noor, and Talah. I told them that some of the names had similarities to names in English and Hebrew, and that many names came from the same source—the Bible or nature—and those were all beautiful names.

We progressed comfortably, and it became clear that some of the girls were extremely bright and very fast learners. Once they overcame their shyness, they were forthcoming and, though speaking in a foreign language, they could be humorous, even playful sometimes, with words or concepts. I appreciated this trait in them, since I had experienced the same challenges myself when trying to express myself in Hebrew. They all seemed eager and would ask me questions at the end of every lesson as I tried to combine the anatomy and physiology together—not treating them as separate entities if I could help it—so that gradually, how the body worked and how it looked came to be meaningful as a combined entity for them.

One day as we sat in our usual room drinking coffee, I said to Noor, "I have a real challenge today because it's time to teach the anatomy and physiology of the pelvic organs and reproductive system. I know that usually it's women—probably their mothers—who would speak to them about this. What should I do? Should you be teaching this rather than I?"

"Why me?" Noor responded. "I am not their instructor of anatomy and physiology. You are! Just go in and teach it like you teach everything else."

"Okay, I just hope this works out," I replied. I entered the room and wrote the title of the day's educational content on the blackboard—"Anatomy of the male reproductive system." They looked up at me, stopping their writing for a moment, then went back to their notebooks and dutifully wrote it down. I took out my chalk and started drawing the penis, using blue and red chalk for veins and arteries. As I turned around, without even taking a look, I could almost see the blushing on their faces, and I had a sense that the temperature of the room had risen by several degrees. They looked furtively at the board, and then back to their notebooks, trying to copy what was on the board. I kept talking and drawing, and the blushing ebbed as I changed focus to the female anatomy, which seemed to cause less consternation. When I came to the physiology and described the sexual and reproductive processes, I could see the blushes and feel the heat again. My drawings were very colorful, and I could see from the books near me that the students were reproducing that color, along with my writing, and drawing, as fast as they could.

As I left, a bit late, and knowing by now that I always had to stop by the ward at the hospital to take care of a few things, I saw Noor. "So?" she inquired.

"I think it went okay—see if you can find out from them—it was quite a class. If their parents knew, they might pull them out of here!" I joked.

By the end of the year, the class had undergone a gradual transformation. Just as we broke for the summer, I noticed that many of the girls had cut their hair a bit—in preparation for working during the summer in the hospital, they said. And they had begun to wear shorter sleeves and shorter skirts. Maybe I was imagining it, but they looked less like rural girls from the West Bank and more like late-adolescent girls and young women from anywhere, not all that different from the girls studying nursing at the Shaare Zedek nursing school. I wished, but knew it premature to ask, that there could be some exchange between the girls from each of the nursing schools.

Another year started, and I shifted to clinical subjects— medicine and surgery—and for the latter, I, myself, needed help from textbooks—but it was basic principles I was teaching so I managed. The girls had become much more mature over the summer and, having had their practical experience, often peppered their questions with references to something that they had seen or heard or witnessed at the hospital where they had been assigned. The time flew by. In the meanwhile, I was arranging to leave for Canada for some postgraduate training. I told Noor that we were looking for a replacement, someone for whom English was the mother tongue. Prior to my leaving, a Canadian whom I had met during my residency in Montreal and who had moved to Israel agreed to take on the position. I knew they were in good hands. I said a warm and tearful good-bye to the class and to Noor, especially.

My one hope was that the school would continue and that these girls would be a legacy to this positive and fulfilling example of cooperation between our peoples. I hoped, too, that somewhere in their memories would remain the wonderful lessons we had learned from each other, just as they stayed within me. Recently, with the power of the Internet, I found the name of a nurse who I thought might have been in that first class. When I contacted her, I received the following e-mail message, "I will never forget my teacher, Dr. Gordon, with his lovely jeans and his shoes which were beige in its color. Yes, I am the one who you are searching after." She wrote me her name and told me she was from Nablus. "You were my teacher in the anatomy and physiology in 1972." The student had lived in many places, including Europe, at the time she wrote to me; she went on to describe to me her marvelous clinical and academic achievements, which included becoming a dean of nursing.

*   *   *

It was likely because of these memories that I had eagerly welcomed the opportunity to visit Qatar and participate in the two academic seminars that would be attended by people from all over the Middle East and the Gulf region. Maybe I would reconnect with a former student or two. However, soon after accepting the invitation, I became concerned because, according to the Qatar national Web site, I could be refused entry because my passport had stamps registering my frequent visits to Israel. My Qatari physician host tried to mollify me by telling me he knew of Israeli guests who had visited the country. Just to be safe, I decided to use my option as a dual Canadian-American citizen, and applied for my entry visa using my American passport. My fears would later turn out to be unfounded: after I returned home and searched the updated Qatar Web sites, I discovered that the previously noted criteria for refusal based on Israeli immigration stamps had been removed.

As the date of the conference neared, I became ambivalent about going, partially because I would be a Jew in an Arabic nation, and partially because I had communication problems with the conference organizers. I had last-minute cold feet because of a ticket mix-up, but decided to go anyway because this was a unique opportunity and an adventure I had long anticipated. My wife Gilda, who I had married in 1982 some years after the breakup of my first marriage with Yael, had a nightmare or two. She was somewhat apprehensive about her Jewish Brooklyn Boy heading to the Persian Gulf. Yet, within a short period after I arrived and was literally whisked through immigration and customs as a VIP, I was immediately struck by the hospitality, the affluence, and generosity of the people.

There was quite a wide range of dress in the conference participants—all of whom came from Muslim countries—which mirrored the range of dress seen in Doha, the country's capital. Many Qataris wore traditional dress—the men in white robes and *guthra* headdresses, and the women in all black *abayas*—some with their faces covered, and some only covering their hair. In contrast, a number of the nonlocal conference delegates wore western clothes, with little of the focus on modesty that appeared to be favored in Qatar. This was brought home to me during a luncheon for the speakers at a fashionable seaside Lebanese-cuisine restaurant.

At the long restaurant table, I was seated next to a Moroccan professor of philosophy with whom I communicated in my broken, but adequate, French. Across the table was a Lebanese English-speaking sociology professor. Both were wearing western-style business suits, rather than Gulf State–style robes and head coverings. Farther down the table was a woman wearing snugly fitting, rhinestone-ornamented black designer jeans and a formfitting, scoop-necked T-shirt. I thought to myself that this is how my then eighteen-year-old daughter would be dressed in a restaurant or pub in Toronto or Tel-Aviv. After the main buffet courses, the two men joined another table and the woman moved opposite me, introducing herself as a Syrian journalist. Her English was flawless, and I could not help but wonder how she could dress the way she did. After some preliminary inquiries about my role at the conference, she asked if she could interview me for her newspaper. I agreed.

She took out her tape recorder, and we embarked on a forty-five-minute interview about the challenges of aging.

We touched on my experiences and challenges as they related to Judaism, Israel, the Middle East, the Gulf States, Western Europe, and North America. She showed nothing but great interest in all that I said. I felt so comfortable with the interview that we ended up speaking about our personal lives, even comparing notes on the raising of adolescents, as we both had adolescent children of comparable ages. We laughingly agreed that teenagers are a major challenge to any parent's mental stability, almost anywhere in the world.

One of the more profound conversations I had on this trip followed two presentations on the medical challenges of adolescents, one by a senior Saudi psychiatrist, and a second by a young Palestinian physician who was studying in Canada. The Saudi psychiatrist suggested that terrorism, including suicide bombing, could be explained by depression resulting in a death wish that might also involve the killing of others deemed to be an enemy. A psychiatrist from Bahrain introduced himself to the Palestinian physician and myself during the coffee break and commented emphatically that the link made by the Saudi psychiatrist between depression and terrorism was absurd. This resulted in an hour and a half of discussion on his perspective of the politics, history, and potential future of the Gulf, the Middle East, and the Arab worlds.

He indicated to me, as I shared my Jewish- and Israeli-related heritage with him, that he believed that terrorism had nothing to do with psychiatric disorders such as depression; rather, it came, in his view, from a misguided understanding of Islam, a very limited view of the regional political realities, as well as a lack of appreciation for the opportunities to create a better and more productive region. I was absolutely mesmerized by this physician who, while wearing traditional Gulf Region dress, spoke so candidly to me of the horror and futility of terrorism, and of the need for the Arab world to fight against it by introducing democracy into its political infrastructure.

"We must stop looking backward, but rather look forward, to succeed in the contemporary world," he said.

He left me almost speechless as he wove his comments and vision, quoted literary sources, and decried the commitment to terror. He recommended prohibiting hateful speech in schools and mosques and proposed a clear separation of religion from the worlds of politics and science. He actually said, "Why are all the speakers praising Allah before they give their presentation? Leave Allah to the mosques and to one's actions. Keep science where it belongs—in the schools and universities and at academic presentations." We wished each other well, and I hoped that his views were more accepted than I had otherwise believed before I came to the conference.

My participation in the conferences was coming to an end. Prior to my flight, I was able to join the speakers and organizers for a last, sumptuous dinner. After receiving good and safe travel wishes from those who had become my academic and conference colleagues, I had a final conversation with the Qatari director of research at Doha University, whose beautiful face was uncovered despite the fact that she wore a traditional black *abaya*. I asked her why she did not cover her face when other married Qatari women did.

She told me that it was her personal choice, and that, when considering marriage, she had told her prospective husband that he would have to accept her as an equal in all respects, and this would include her being able to face the world with her face open to it at all times. She implied that being open to the world and having the world witness who she was, with all her facial expressions and their meanings, was very important to her feeling of full participation in the world of progress, scientific inquiry, and human interaction.

By visiting Qatar, I, too, had the opportunity to open myself to a whole other world and have that world witness the person I am. This had been a unique opportunity for me. After only a few days in the country and a few conversations with my counterparts, I realized that there is as much variety of opinion, contradiction, and modern thought in the Arabic Gulf and Middle East as there is in North America, Israel, and the rest of the Western world. To travel to the Arab world and to see myself as a peer among professionals who dressed and spoke in ways that were foreign to me, and then to break bread with them, sharing conversations and our lives, was an extraordinary experience that offered me far more than I ever could have imagined it would.

Chapter 12
Getting It Right

"I understand that Yoel is leaving."

"That's right," I said to Steve, my CEO. "He is going to Israel to live. I am not surprised." Without any formal training in ethics, Yoel had done an excellent job in forming an ethics committee and getting its operations off the ground, initiating the same process at Baycrest that most hospitals in Canada were undertaking in the late 1990s. "So who is going to chair the ethics committee?" asked Steve. I explained that I did not know, but would put out feelers to members of the department who I thought might be interested. (As head of medical services, staffing committee positions was one of my responsibilities.) Two weeks and many e-mails later, I wrote to Steve, "I will take it on for the year until I can find someone to do it. Everyone says they are either too busy or do not feel comfortable doing it. I'll get some advice about what to do."

"Fine," was the reply, in keeping with the way Steve operated: Got a problem? Get someone to solve it!

I spoke to Yoel, the geriatrician in question, whom I had recruited right out of training, a lovely, sweet, clever man who was quite religious and brought that perspective to the committee. The religious perspective was important for a Jewish institution like Baycrest—but alone was not enough as we were part of the secular, publicly funded healthcare system. He filled me in on the progress of the committee during his period as chair. For further advice, I contacted Dr. Fred Lowy, with whom I had worked a few years before on a major project for the provincial government, after which he had taken over as director of the fairly new University of Toronto Joint Centre for Bioethics.

"What should I do to take this on, Fred? The only thing I know about medical ethics is from a book I reviewed some years ago for the CMAJ (the *Canadian Medical Association Journal*)—and that was pretty rudimentary—plus the fact that I studied Philosophy 101 at Brooklyn College in the late 1950s. I loved it but, after all, what real use are Plato, Aristotle, Kant, and Kierkegaard?" I could hear Fred laughing on the other end of the phone.

"Start coming down to the Joint Centre on Wednesday afternoons and listen to the presentations—the 4:00 PM to 5:00 PM presentation is open to the public—and, if you are interested, we can allow you to sit in on the 3:00 PM to 4:00 PM, which is for the postgrad students in ethics. Then we can talk about how to go about doing this. I will also give you a few books to read."

A year later found me mulling around the courtyard at Georgetown University waiting for the orientation to a week-long intensive program on medical ethics for people like myself, novices in the field who were going to either sit on or chair ethics committees. (Most of the students were from the United States, but a few of us were from Canada.) The year had passed, and I was still unable to find anyone to take on the role of chair, and, in the meantime, had begun to enjoy the Wednesday sessions.

"Steve," I said, "I will stay on as chair as long as you help me get educated in the field. Here is the application for a weeklong course in Georgetown. Pay for it and my travel, and I will give you at least another year and then we can see." "Done!" he replied, signing the registration form and the check requisition right there on the spot.

The course was the beginning of a new career direction for me. I listened to some of the great names in contemporary medical ethics—Beauchamp, Childress, Thomasma, and Pellegrino. They were spellbinding speakers, but the best part was the students. They were from everywhere and every background—doctors, nurses, lawyers, and administrators. We argued and joked, ate and drank together, and I came back feeling I could take on anything that might come to the ethics committee. After a few meetings and some explorations, it became clear that what I had learned was merely the introduction to a very long story, and that the group of volunteers on the committee and I had a lot to do. An eager postgraduate administration student was assigned to me that year, and, with his assistance, we put together the framework of our committee as I continued to attend the seminars.

After another year, Peter Singer, the new director of the Joint Centre, called me in one day after a session and said, "I think, if you are going to do this seriously, you have to get your master's degree in ethics."

"You're kidding, of course! Why can't I just continue doing this the way I am now?" Even as I said the words I realized, myself, that he was right. I had been thinking already that I should take on the study of ethics at a more serious level. It took a year to arrange, as there was no formal program at the university at the time designed for working people who wanted to complete their master's on a part-time basis, but Dr. Cathy Whiteside, the incumbent director of the medical faculty's research institute, figured out a way for me to do it. So I embarked on the program, one course at a time, without having to give up any of my work at Baycrest. Once again, I learned to study at night, write papers, and do presentations.

Two years later, I completed the course work and, two years after that, a thesis focusing on resource allocation in government-supported drug programs around the United States and Canada with attention to the coverage of Viagra, which had just come onto the market. The day I presented my defense, the bulb went out on the projector—there were no spares—and it was snowing outside so heavily that one of the panel members could not make it. Nevertheless, we were able to hook up my presentation to a conference call, and we got through it. I was awarded a master of science in medical ethics.

*   *   *

When I think back to the difficult cases of my long medical career, some of the most complex ones, invariably, would now be framed as ethical challenges rather than clinical conundrums, although the latter, of course, still occurred. I recall when, as a medical resident in Jerusalem, I ran the ICU, and a young Russian patient was brought in with a ruptured cerebral aneurysm. This was in the days before CT scans and likely successful surgery for such catastrophes. The hospital had one of the few sophisticated respirators in Jerusalem, so he was on it in a semicomatose state for weeks with everyone— the staff and his family—waiting for his recovery. With time, the likelihood of this happening became increasingly remote. He developed one infection after another. We knew he would die, but his mother and sister were by his side day in and day out; there was no way, it seemed, that we could discontinue what was becoming futile treatment. His death was horrible because, in essence, he was neurologically dead and then had a cardiac arrest. As the family hovered around, we tried what we knew to be fruitless cardiac massage, but, when it was clear that it was over, they started to scream in Hebrew and Russian for us to continue. "You can't stop—Sasha, please, Sasha—

you can't stop, doctor, please keep trying." It was an awful scene, typical of many in which I played a part at the time, thinking only in terms of the clinical outcome to a life-and-death situation without regard to the ethical issues involved.

Later on in my career, we did begin to examine such situations through an ethical lens, using the new language of ethics with its autonomy, beneficence, non–malfeasance, and justice—the so-called "Georgetown mantra"—as if by using these terms the poignancy of the human tragedies that we faced could more easily be managed. From the first case presented formally to our ethics committee until now, much of my latter career interest has become focused on the complexities of the human condition and the interface between medicine and the ethics of decision-making.

*   *   *

"Please stop the feeding tube—we made a terrible mistake!" These words were said in the hallway by a physician who had once been a colleague during an earlier period of my career. He was referring to his mother, now a patient at Baycrest on one of the complex units. She was semicomatose from a stroke, and had a feeding tube in place.

"George, let us arrange for a meeting with you and your family and the staff on the unit to discuss this. A hallway is not a good place to deal with this, okay?" I expected to hear within a few days that a meeting had been called, but there was no message, so I assumed the situation had been resolved. The day before I was leaving for a conference in Chicago, I received word that an urgent meeting about the mother with the feeding tube was requested late that afternoon with the doctor, his sister, and their spouses.

"Michael, we realize we made a terrible error when we agreed to put the tube in when she was at the hospital. She had recovered pretty well from the other stroke, you know. Sure, this was a bigger one, but we hoped she would make some recovery. She has not, and now we can't bear to watch her. She hardly opens her eyes, and we don't think she recognizes anyone." We went around and asked all the members of the family how they felt, and they all concurred.

The head nurse was a bit puzzled as she said that Rose had not deteriorated since she had come in; in fact, she was quite stable and not suffering at all. "Why now, all of a sudden?" she wanted to know.

"It is not all of a sudden," Julie, the daughter, replied. "It is just that we have struggled with this for months and realize that we have to make a decision. We hoped maybe she would get sick or develop an infection, and then we could just let nature takes its course, but that has not happened. We really believe that, if she were able to speak for herself, she would never agree to this."

The nurse's face revealed some consternation, but she did not say anything more. The family stepped out for a few minutes as the small group of staff that remained, and I, as chair of the ethics committee, conferred. I reminded them, "The family does have the legal right to discontinue treatment. If they believe that is what she would have wanted, there is nothing more to say."

"Don't they need a living will stating just that?" asked the head nurse.

"Not really; if there is one, that may help, but if the family believes this is what their mother would have wanted—and they are the substitute decision-makers—then that is enough. I will arrange for the order to be written in the morning."

The head nurse replied, "I don't think Dr. Klein will write it. I heard him say earlier today when he found out about the meeting that he could not write such an order for personal moral reasons."

"Well, if he won't, then I will write it in the morning after

I speak to the staff on the morning shift. I am leaving in the afternoon for a few days in Chicago."

There were some nurses, a social worker, and the dietician at the morning meeting the next day. "The family wants to discontinue the tube feeding," I advised them. "We discussed it last night, and they all seem to agree. They feel strongly that she would not have wanted to be kept alive like this."

"I don't understand—how can they just do that? She is no worse than she was—we have really provided excellent care. This is like killing her. Are you sure our College of Nurses (the regulatory council of the nursing profession in Ontario) accepts a thing like that?" That was from a senior nurse, though I could see nodding from the other nurses in the group.

The dietician countered, "The College of Dieticians of Ontario certainly allows for patients to stop using tube feeding if they choose, or if their substitute decision-makers choose."

"But you do not provide the day-to-day care," another nurse piped in. "To us, it feels like murder. I don't care what the law says, I can only tell you how I feel."

"I know how it must feel to all of you who have provided such wonderful care," I interjected, "but the family is allowed to do this. You have all had patients or families who have refused tube feeds, right?" There was nodding all around. "Well, had the family refused six months ago, she would have died then. They gave it a try to see if she would recover—and she didn't. Isn't it better to have given her the chance?"

"Well, it just does not feel good after all those months of nursing care," replied the nurse. "She does not have even one pressure ulcer on her!"

I went out of the room, found the chart, and wrote the order to discontinue tube feeding and to focus on comfort measures, with mouth care and other excellent nursing procedures. I left that night, as planned, for Chicago. I heard nothing the next day, but that evening there was an e-mail from the clinical nurse specialist covering the unit. "The nurses are in an uproar. They say they cannot take care of her with this order—and they are going to complain to the college that they have been forced to compromise their standards of care." I wrote back that they could do whatever they wanted with their college, but they could not withhold care that had been ordered. The nurse responded that the doctor on duty had not actually canceled the order I had written, but was verbally supporting their position; and, in the meantime, tube feeding and all other care was being provided. Apparently, one of the nurses had asked the son how he and his family could do such a thing, and the son had complained to the head nurse about being spoken to in that manner. Early the next morning, I called the physician who was running the palliative care program at Baycrest and explained the situation (palliative care focuses on easing the physical symptoms and addressing the psychosocial needs in individuals in their last stage of life when it is agreed that the underlying disease can no longer be treated in any beneficial manner). "I know this is not the way we should normally address this issue, but because I am away and cannot speak to the group directly, would you agree to transfer the patient to your unit and allow her to die in peace? Ask your team first, though, if they will have any problem with the process that has been requested and ordered by me."

He replied in a reassuring way. "I do not have to ask the team. I know for sure they would view this as part of an acceptable framework for the terminal phase of a palliative care plan. I will arrange to transfer her today."

I communicated to the head nurse, the clinical nurse specialist, and the attending physician with the following: "Under the circumstances, and because I am not there to speak directly to the staff, I have arranged for the patient to be transferred to palliative care in order to meet her end-of-life needs. Please inform the family. I will be back on the weekend, but am going away again at the first of the week. I will try to come in and see how things are going."

I visited the patient (whose daughter was with her) on Saturday morning. She had been transferred Friday morning and was comfortable. "Has she responded to your being here?" I asked.

"Not at all, not since the evening before she was transferred. We think she is comfortable. The nurses are wonderful. I know her nurses from the other floor were very upset—they have been with her for almost six months and are very attached to her—but we had to make this decision. Thanks for helping us. How much longer do you think we will have her?"

"I would think maybe five or six more days or so." I left town the next day, and three days later received an e-mail that she had died, peacefully without any problems.

On my return, we had a debriefing with the nursing staff and other members of the team. "The College said we had to follow the request of the surrogate and that we would not be deemed to be acting unprofessionally if we did so," said one of the nurses.

"The College of Social Workers said the same," was the reply from the unit's social worker.

"I know that the College of Physicians has the same type of policy," I added, "because that is what the law says: a person, or a person's substitute, can refuse, withdraw, or withhold treatment if the person is capable of making such a decision or if the substitute believes that is what the person would have wanted."

"But it came so suddenly," lamented the nurse. "It was such a shock after all those months of looking after her, with never a word, not a hint."

"I wish we could have spoken to the family so that we could hear from them what they thought was happening and why they made the decision," said another. "If we had, I am sure we would have been able to fulfill their wishes. This way,

she died on another ward among strangers. We knew her—
what a shame it happened this way."

I could see that many of the nurses were upset. "I think
you are right; it was a shame it happened so fast. I will do
my best in the future to make sure the staff has more lead
time, if possible, and that you can hear directly from a family
member what they are experiencing and the decisions they
have made. Hopefully, that way, you will all feel comfortable
doing something which I know is very hard for you." They all
nodded, and the meeting ended.

*   *   *

Feeding tubes are one of the contentious issues in long-
term care ethics because, for so many, using a feeding tube is
equated with love and devotion, just as administering food
and drink are. The issue has evolved to being one of whether
artificial nutrition and hydration is equivalent to eating and
drinking and whether not using—or stopping—a feeding tube
is the same as not giving someone food and water. It is often
a controversial issue—but no less so is the issue of cardiac
resuscitation—known as CPR.

"He said he spoke to the rabbi that the family used to go to
when the mother was well and living in the community. The
rabbi says, no matter what, we have to provide CPR. So, that
is what he wants." One of the hospital physicians was relating
to me what the son of a patient had said at a recent family
meeting. "I explained to him the protocols and guidelines for
CPR and DNR (do not resuscitate) at Baycrest," the physician
said, "but the son said he would speak to the rabbi and this is
what he came back with. It does not fit into our guidelines, so
I had another meeting with the son who was accompanied by
his sister and the head nurse, advising the two of them that,
if the event is not witnessed and the mother is *found* without
vital signs—especially if it is likely that it has been some time

since she was last seen—then we would not perform CPR." Their response was, 'We demand that you do it. It is our legal right and part of our religion—and your responsibility is to respect our religious rights.' I tried to explain that this has nothing to do with religion, but that the policy was developed based on the realities of end-of-life events and the limited possibilities of CPR. They told me they did not care and would complain to the newspapers and the government and the CEO."

I said I would meet with the son and daughter and the head nurse together so that each could hear the other. In the meantime, I printed out a number of important and well-thought-out articles on the subject that demonstrated the limits of CPR in the long-term care of the elderly—and often frail—population, as well as some articles from Jewish literature. For good measure, I added the codes of ethics governing nurses and doctors that justified the limits to which we should go. Desecrating the body of a person who was clearly dead was not something the nursing staff felt comfortable with, quite rightly insisting that they knew the difference between someone who had just died—or arrested—and one who had been dead for a while.

We met, though the meeting started off with a tense undertone. "You must know that we only want the best for your mother," I said. "If there is an intervention that we do not think we should apply, it is for a very good and well-thought-out reason. In fact, the easiest thing we could do is just agree to call a 'code' on her, do CPR until the ambulance comes, and then let her die in an emergency room in the company of people who do not know her and who, in all honesty, probably do not care much what the outcome of their efforts may be. After all, for them she is simply a very old, demented lady from a nursing home, not a member of an extended family, which is what she is to us."

The daughter thought for a while and replied, "I want

the best for my mother and do not want to be responsible for her death. She has been through so much—she survived the Holocaust, you know—and I could not live with myself if there were something that should have been done that I did not do." Her brother nodded in agreement. "And the rabbi said that, according to Jewish law, I had to do it."

I explained the studies on CPR in the elderly in long-term care facilities and gave the two of them copies of some of the articles on the subject. But knowing it would be more meaningful for them, I also added articles from rabbinical scholars on CPR that explained the law, agreeing that there could be limits to when attempts might be undertaken. I also showed them policies and statements from our various professional codes of ethics about respect for the person—dead and alive—so they would know that, in the face of a person who was truly believed to be dead, it would be unacceptable for a nurse to undertake CPR, and that no one could order a nurse to do so without risk of censure by the regulatory body.

"But, most importantly, do you really want your mother's last experience on earth after so much suffering to be a most undignified, and possibly painful, experience that, at the same time, will not provide her with any semblance of survival?" I prodded. "The very few who manage to survive CPR often die within a short period, often without ever having gained consciousness. Is that really want you think she would have wanted—which is the main question—or even what you would want for your mother, which is the secondary question."

A few days later, they agreed to our framework; likewise, we agreed to provide CPR in the event that we witnessed a loss of vital signs. This followed professional protocols, yet satisfied their need to feel that everything that could be done would be done.

*   *   *

"I need help with the son, who is a doctor and has just flown in from out of town. He is upsetting the whole family with what he thinks the living will means."

The attending physician had been struggling with the family of an elderly male patient whose blood disease had taken a very malignant turn. The struggle was over whether or not he should be given any further blood transfusions. They had agreed to give a few more units. Each transfusion had a beneficial effect for only a few days until the hemoglobin fell and he became symptomatic again. The attending physician felt that, according to the written living will on record, no heroic measures should be taken, and only comfort care should be provided in the end-of-life situation. Previously, the family had agreed that, after the most recent transfusion, his discomfort and shortness of breath would be treated symptomatically and all efforts should focus on ensuring him some comfortable last days and as quiet a death as possible.

"This is not acceptable," the physician son insisted, even though his mother was the designated substitute decision-maker, and, because the patient was quite somnolent most of the time, could not make his own decisions. The mother was now clearly deferring to her physician son whereas, prior to his arrival, she had been willing to listen to, and discuss the course with, her daughter and youngest son, both of whom lived in the same city as the parents. Her daughter, in fact, had been closest to the patient and had often been involved in his care over the past few years. "Giving blood is not heroic," said the son. "It is symptomatic treatment. It would be inhuman and immoral to deprive him of such treatment."

The attending physician, very conscious of the patient's course as he had looked after him for over a year, felt that the patient would not have wanted to have his life dragged out like this. When he brought this into the discussion, the son replied, "You could not know our father as we do, and, even though I have been away for the past year—other than one short visit a few months ago—I know my father; and I know medicine, so the decision is quite clear—give him as much blood as often as needed to keep him comfortable and alive."

The attending physician was very upset with the son's approach. He felt that he, as the patient's physician, understood the patient well for they had spoken often over the past year. Should the patient have been able to indicate his wishes, he likely would have asked to have the blood transfusions discontinued. The physician also felt that to use such a scarce resource as blood for someone who was clearly in the process of dying was not just patently unfair to all who donated blood in good faith, but also to those in need of the blood (even though there was no indication that there was a shortage of blood in the system at the time these events were taking place).

A meeting was held between the staff, the family, and me, in my role as ethicist. I began, "Why do you think your father wrote what he did in his living will about being allowed to die comfortably and not being subjected to heroics? Also, why do you think your father spoke to the doctor about his wishes all these months if he could not count on him to act in his best interests and as he would have wanted?" I continued, "Is there anywhere that he indicated that he would want his life prolonged in this manner when he is not going to gain consciousness and literally lives from one transfusion to the next, with the day in between being more and more uncomfortable? The doctor would like to treat him in a palliative fashion, with medication to deal with his shortness of breath so that his last days can be comfortable. This transfusing over and over again is really interfering with that approach."

There was a pause as the physician son looked at his mother, the attending physician, the nurses, and, lastly, at me. "Could we agree to give him blood transfusions for another week, and not give him any potent analgesics that will make him sleepy, to see if he might rally and wake up so that we can all have a few last words with him?" the son pleaded. He had tears in his eyes. It was becoming clear why he was pursuing this particular course. He had not seen his father for a number of months, and the way things would likely go without the attempt he was suggesting meant there would be no chance for him to say good-bye to his father.

The attending physician looked at him and said, "Sure, we could do that; let us say up to six units of blood? That may give us up to three weeks, depending on how quickly his hemoglobin falls. As long as he is not expressing severe pain or shortness of breath, I can hold off on the opiates and other such drugs."

The mother took her son's hand and said, "We can hope he will wake up enough to see you one last time. If not, I know how much he loved you and always knew how much you cared about him." Three weeks and six units of blood passed by, and the patient did not wake up. We stopped the transfusions, and, as he became short of breath, treated him for his symptom, with the son and his mother almost always by his side. They had come to accept the reality of the situation and the limits of care, as well as the importance of trying to heed the wishes of those we love.

*   *   *

These latter years of my career, accompanied by a more pronounced role and involvement in ethics, have helped me to become increasingly aware of just how much family and staff members alike struggle with the challenge of doing the right thing for those we care for. Professionals and family members share in a very difficult decision-making process. Those of us who are the professionals know, or may have already experienced in our own lives, what it is like to be on the other side of the bed as a family member. Having experienced both sides of the situation myself has certainly helped me to appreciate the enormous challenges, tenderness, poignancy, and trepidation that we all face in these most difficult life-ending and life-defining situations.

This type of work has been one of the most profoundly interesting, challenging, and rewarding chapters of my professional story. I feel humbled and privileged to have played a part in the many life-defining moments of so many people and their families. They looked to me for care and advice and—from time to time—wisdom. And while wisdom may be most desired when a family is making such difficult decisions, in all humility, I recognize that it is the hardest attribute to come by.

Chapter 13

Personal Challenges and the Second Time Around

In most families, there are wonderful experiences and exchanges of love, acts of self-sacrifice, and the important elements that help us grow into the persons that we become. The losses that always inevitably must occur in families are never forgotten, with some being part of the expected "seasons" of life, a metaphor often contained in the eulogies over the dead at funerals of many faiths. The loss of my mother was very sad, not just because she was such a wonderful person and she died before Talia and Eytan had enough years to really get to know her—and she enjoyed being with them so much—but also because she suffered during her final, dying days. Of the many lessons I learned from her hospitalization and dying process, the most important was that being a son who is a geriatrician did not provide any major advantage when it came to dealing with illness and, ultimately, death. Of course I could ask the right questions and, at times, *demand* interventions that a lay person might not have known about, but, in the end, her death was unfortunately one of pain and suffering, which all the expressions of dismay by myself and my sister Diti did relatively little to ameliorate. What the experience did give me, though, was a greater understanding and appreciation of the process of illness and the struggles of sons and daughters trying to cope with the unknown or the known, especially when the latter is devoid of hope.

The other thing my mother's illness and death taught me was how important it is for sons and daughters to tell their parents how much they mean to them and how wonderful they are more often than is generally the case. As I sat by my mother's bedside on the medical floor of Coney Island Hospital in Brooklyn, I wished I had been less critical of her for her personal failings, and, instead, had simply told her just what a wonderful mother she had been. Throughout those last days of her life, I held her hand and spoke to her even though she was supposedly in coma. Following her death, I promised myself that I would tell my father what a great father he was to me, not just when he was ill, but every time I saw him.

The first occasion came some months after my mother's death while he was still struggling to cope alone in the small bungalow in Brooklyn. I had come down for a visit and, at one point just prior to my returning home to Toronto, I said, "Daddy, I just want to tell you what a wonderful father you have always been and how much I owe to you." He looked at me for a few moments before speaking. I had never said anything like that to him before.

"Is there something wrong? Did you get a bad report from the doctor that I do not know about? Am I dying?"

I looked at him and said, "No," and started to laugh, and then he started to laugh. "I just want to make sure that you know how I feel about you."

"You don't have to say it. I know it!" was his reply.

I could not implement all that easily the many lessons I learned from being a geriatrician, nor did Diti's social work role help her that much either when it came to making the difficult decisions we were faced with when, as my father lived alone in the Brooklyn bungalow he had shared with our mother, his health began to fail. Finally, after over a year of trying to convince him to try moving to Canada, where I knew I and my wife Gilda and two children could provide excellent and loving care to him with access to a wide array of services, we ultimately told him he would have to move to Chicago to be close to Diti. He had refused Canada, even after I secured immigrant status for him, because he was afraid the "taxes were too high" and that he would lose his driver's license. All the explanations about the reality of income tax at his stage of life and the driving situation were not enough to change his decision to let his entry permit lapse.

The discussion that finally led to his reluctant agreement to move to Chicago for a "trial" was precipitated by a birthday celebration where we joined him and his sister and brother-in-law for a dinner at a well-known restaurant in Sheepshead Bay, not far from his home. After the dinner, while the other guests had gone to the washrooms before leaving, he turned to Diti, who was sitting with him, and asked, "How did I get here?" When we took him home, we were shocked to find the house a disaster, with dishes piled in the sink, food everywhere, his bed clearly not made for weeks, and pill boxes from over-the-counter sleeping medications and, most telling, a half-finished bottle of gin on the dresser which he had been using to help him sleep. He had been self-medicating because of back pain and difficulty sleeping. There were mouse droppings all along the living room floor, especially against the wall near the dining room table. He was sitting, and we faced him.

Diti started, "Daddy, we cannot leave you in Brooklyn like this. Things are falling apart. The bathroom is hardly functioning, and the place is filthy. There are mouse droppings all over the place."

He looked up at her and then me and said, "They are quite entertaining." He looked down at his hands folded in front of him and to our surprise said, "Okay, I will go—but only to try it out. Do not sell the house." We were shocked and surprised and relieved.

Within a week, Diti had secured a place for a three-month trial in an older retirement home near where she lived. Two weeks later, I came down to help him pack up so that she could drive him there. She reported the trip as being an experience she would not want to do again, but, nevertheless, they had had some good laughs. During the long drive, Diti would repeatedly ask, as she approached a rest stop, if Dad had to use the washroom. He would reply no, only to tell her, as soon as they passed the turnoff, that he did have to urinate. Diti learned quickly to just stop at every rest stop she came to and take him in for a "prophylactic pee." At the motel where they stayed overnight, he asked if she wanted to go gambling. He thought it was a "pretty swanky place" and therefore must be a casino. At the beginning of the trip, Diti had designated him as navigator since he had driven many times from New York to Chicago, but she quickly learned that his directional abilities were not always accurate so, although he continued to give directions, she followed the map without his always realizing it.

Dad settled in to the Oak Park Arms. It was a temporary arrangement, and, with some readjustments of his medications by a geriatrician colleague of mine, his mind improved a great deal, and he began to reevaluate his living situation, only agreeing to stay after a month had passed when he was told that we had prepaid for three months and would lose the money. For a Depression survivor like himself, this was too much for even him to swallow. So he reluctantly stayed on, with his car sitting unused because "we had to get local insurance" for him, a protective ploy that he did not question. One night, Diti got the phone call. Dad could not move his bowels and was in pain. He thought he should go to the hospital. She went over and slept on the extra bed in the alcove in his room. In the meanwhile, she plied him with yogurt, All Bran, and suppositories until, at four in the morning, he had the necessary movement, and, with great relief, went to sleep. In the morning, he acknowledged, in his rather dramatic way, that she had "saved his life" and told her to "sell the house." She called me with the story, and we contacted our neighbor Walter, a real estate broker, to put it on the market. A month later, we were both at the house to clean it up.

"Why don't we just get a dumpster and pour everything in the house into it?" I humorously asked.

"You never know what we might find. They saved everything, and I think we have to see what there is," replied Diti as we worked out a strategy to go through each room and classify and sort what could go, what had to be looked over, and what we had to save to be looked at some other time. (I have heard this story over the years from many of the children of my patients, and knew that one day it would happen to us.) Diti was right. We found treasures of information about our parents' lives, and had many a good laugh—and many a cry—over some of the old letters and documents that were stored in the most unpredictable places. I retrieved every letter I had written to my parents from medical school, and now have them stored in my house for my children to dispose of when the time comes, unless I get around to going through them beforehand. I learned much about my father's accomplishments during the war when he worked as a civilian engineer for the U.S. Department of Defense. Some time later in Chicago, when I read to him a letter of commendation from his commanding officer for his work on the "night vision project," his reply was, "Oh, yeah, he was a very nice man." He did not comment at all on the nature of his own obviously groundbreaking work on what eventually became the infrared nighttime vision devices used by armies all over the world.

One of the most poignant experiences we had was finding a typed letter to my maternal grandfather written in my mother's name (which we assumed someone else had typed for her as we knew or believed that she did not type). It was begging him to return to the family after he had left his wife and two adolescent children. This plea for him to return was full of love as well as of his family's pain at his leaving. We knew that he did not return, and it was not until after our grandmother died that he came back into the family. All my childhood years, I had thought of him as an ogre. He had left my grandmother, this wonderful woman with whom I shared a bedroom along with my sister in our very small Brighton Beach apartment. I had learned from my grandmother about Jewish life in the small village in Lithuania where she originated, and her struggles as a seamstress in the early years of the nonunionized garment industry in New York. Without my realizing it, Grandmother had a profound influence on my life and, I believe, ultimately, my career path, and her estranged husband, whom I had never met, was to me the embodiment of evil.

About a year after her death, he arrived and entered the living room of the same apartment I had shared with my grandmother. I was expecting the worst. Yet, within an hour, I was enchanted by him and realized that my love for photography probably had some biological connection as he, too, was a serious amateur photographer. After he died, I appropriated his Nikkormat, an exact duplicate of the camera I had acquired toward the end of my medical school training and the indestructible mainstay of my cameras, having replaced the pre–Second World War Zeiss Contax 2A. I still own all of them, even though I have replaced my film models with newer digital cameras. Sometime later we met Clara, the woman for whom he had left my grandmother, who also was repatriated into our family network, although my mother's brother Saul, bitter and unforgiving, rejected both of them until the end of their lives and his. The irony of it all is that, after my grandfather died, as Clara became ill and frail and eventually house- and then bed-bound, it was my mother who initially cared for her directly until she required a hired caregiver, who was with her until her dying day. That same caregiver ended up looking after my mother during her last days in hospital, and the circle of love and devotion, despite the undulations of relationships and connections, remained connected.

We emptied as much as we could for garbage pickup; the house was strewn with more than sixty green garbage bags to throw out. There was just one problem: the limit of garbage pickup from an individual house was three bags. We asked Walter, who lived in the neighborhood, for advice, thinking there must be an alternative method for larger amounts.

"No problem," replied Walter with a sly smile. "No one on the street throws out three bags of garbage. Tonight we will distribute the bags up and down the block so everyone will have the honor of contributing to the cleanup of your house. What we cannot place, we will distribute among the many dumpsters of the apartment houses in the neighborhood."

That night, we dragged green garbage bags and put one or two of them next to the one or two bags already put out by the occupants of the small bungalows that lined my parents' street. We managed to get rid of the bulk of the sixty bags, giving an unusually bizarre appearance to the street for its trash collection. Early in the morning, I went out to see if the garbagemen would load all the bags—and they did! What they thought, we never knew. Walter loaded the last few bags into his old Buick, and the two of us roamed the neighborhood, looking at the back of apartment buildings for dumpsters that had room for a few more of my parents' belongings and papers. Walter said as I thanked him, "These are among the many lessons I learned in Russia; sharing one's garbage with neighbors was a very popular activity."

Months later, the house was empty as my father had agreed to stay in Chicago. Walter had his second "honor"—selling the house to another Russian immigrant to Brighton Beach, another added to a growing population of émigrés of which the community already had its fair share. My father was now a permanent resident of Oak Park, Illinois, and a willing occupant of the Oak Park Arms Retirement Home.

My relationship with my sister and parents had always been very close. What with my living overseas from the age of nineteen, and traveling a great deal, much of our relationship was long-distance, but we always managed a great closeness when it came to affection. My parents supported all my personal endeavors and hoped always, as parents do, that my marital and family situation would be happy and stable. That goal was a bit circuitous and complex, but, no matter what happened in my personal and family life, they were always there for me and did whatever was necessary to provide me with emotional support. As is often the case with grandparents, they relished their grandchildren, were interested in whatever was happening in our lives, and, when things were especially challenging because of the disruptions in my first marriage, they were there with support and love for their beloved grandchildren.

When a marriage dies, it is often the case that it is only in looking back that it becomes clear that the relationship had been ailing for a long time. So was the case with my marriage to Yael. When were the first signs of its failing state? Of course, looking back, it's easier to see the indicators, some earlier than others, but such clarity of vision is only gained after the fact with hindsight. The years in Israel were difficult but also wonderfully challenging with many satisfactions. Our two children, Neta and Amir, were born, I became acclimatized to a new country, and Yael completed her bachelor's degree.

There were challenges and problems as exist with any couple, but especially so for us given the strains of an immigrant experience in a country always under internal and external stress. One of the problems with relationships in Israel is that, with pressure all the time from wars and threats of war, it almost seems selfish to dwell on the difficulties of interpersonal relationships. I would actually say at times that it seemed selfish to be concerned about problems over understanding or communication when every day on the news some real or potential existential threat loomed on the horizon. Certainly, during my military service, when real threats did exist, it would have seemed ridiculous to bring up some of the issues on which interpersonal relationships are built. We took all the normal steps to enrich our commitment to each other by having a family, on the common assumption that children bring couples closer together, and we both really did want to have a family. Neta was born in 1971 just toward the end of my military service. The wives of the officers on the base were constantly giving advice to Yael on proper infant care. It was a very warm and caring environment despite the loud sounds of jets overhead from time to time, though these did not seem to disturb Neta at all. Amir was born in 1973, just a few months before we left for Toronto with the intention of my pursuing further medical training and Yael's undertaking some postgraduate education.

The move to Toronto was not easy. There were adjustment difficulties with two small children to deal with as well as our own acclimatization. The outbreak of the Yom Kippur War on October 6, 1973, added a new dimension of tension as we both had to contend with the fact that, with Israel's fate at risk, we were safe in Canada and not in danger in Israel. My parents came to visit to offer help with the children. As for the war, I was glued to the television.

"You will see, the counterattack will occur soon," I kept saying as the reports of the Egyptian move across the Suez Canal and into the Sinai Peninsula proceeded for the first few days without any apparent ability on Israel's part to halt it. I felt a pang of guilt.

I should be there with my unit. They need me; they need everyone, I thought, but, of course, we were committed to our challenges in Canada and could not return. The turn of the tide of events in the war took what seemed like an eternity to occur, and only much later in time did it become clear to me—and to many other Jews—just how close Israel had come to a terrible outcome, even possible defeat.

Life began to take on some semblance of normality. Yael started working part-time in a physician's office. With my extra work moonlighting in an emergency room and a loan from my parents, we moved from an eighteenth-floor apartment—which terrified me because of our active two-year-old—to a townhouse in the same, and by now, familiar area. While I was completing the residency year in nuclear medicine—knowing full well that I would likely not be pursuing it—my moonlighting reminded me just how much I loved the specialty of internal medicine. Neither of us expressed a desire to return to Israel in the immediate future. I passed my Royal College specialty exams in medicine and was recruited to Baycrest and Mt. Sinai concurrently, as wonderful a position as I could imagine. It was hard to believe that we had overcome the difficulties of acclimatizing to a new country, a new job with many examinations, and other hurdles. I became more optimistic about the future.

Years passed; the children seemed to flourish, and my work was more wonderful than I could have imagined. I became more involved in teaching and seemed to have excelled in that field. By chance, I was exposed to television through a contact from work, ultimately resulting in a weekly spot on a CBC television series on health. With the ongoing preparation of scripts for the show, I wondered about putting them together into a book and started playing with that idea, finding that my lifelong interest in writing helped bring ideas to fruition. I submitted the manuscript to thirty-two publishers and received thirty rejections.

I did some investigation on the first publisher that accepted and found that the company did not seem to be of a sufficiently high quality. While I was at a lecture one afternoon, my pager went off, and the switchboard gave me a long-distance number to call—collect.

"This is Frank Taylor from Chiltern Books. I just read your manuscript, and I love it. Can you come to New York to discuss the next steps? It needs a lot of work before we can move forward."

I called my best friend from university days, who was now a professor of English. "Chuck, I think I have a publisher in New York. He wants me to come down to see him. Can I stay with you?" I knew the last question was rhetorical, as I always stayed in his spacious Upper West Side apartment.

Frank was sitting in his Upper East Side apartment where I had been invited to meet and discuss the project. He put his hand on my knee and started to talk about the book.

"You have a great book here, but turn it around so that, rather than being didactic and explaining things, you *talk* to your reader. Use the words *you* and *we* and *him* and *her*—same content ... but make it a conversation."

I replied. "I wrote this because of my television series," and explained the format of the "visit to the doctor."

"Exactly! You talked to the viewers ... now talk to the readers! By the way, can you do it in three months?"

As I was leaving the apartment, I noted some lovely black-and-white photographs on the wall, many of Frank and what appeared to be his family. They seemed to reflect a rich and unconventional life. He was a wonderful editor to work with and largely responsible for the success of the book.

While in New York, I had a chance to speak to Chuck and fill him in on my life in Toronto. We had been very close since university days; while I was in medical school, he did his Navy service and then spent a year in Edinburgh, which gave us a chance to share some wonderful experiences and travel together. We had been best men at each other's weddings.

His had broken up recently, and he was still in the throes of figuring out what to do.

"Things are not good at home," I revealed to him. I did not have any confidants in Toronto other than a therapist I had started going to in order to help me through my marital difficulties. We had tried various attempts at dealing with the problems, but, ultimately, it became clear that our marriage could not be sustained. We decided we would have to find as good a way as possible to bring it to an end, with the best arrangements possible for the children. In the meanwhile, I was compelled by the promise I had made to Frank Taylor and my compulsion to finish my first book, so continued to work on the manuscript despite the problems in my personal life. Because it was the days before computers, the secretary from work whom I hired to do my typing in her free time had a considerable amount of work to do—three carbon copies of a retyped manuscript—but with her IBM Selectric, her deft hands, and impeccable typing skills, she had the edited manuscript ready three months later, as planned. After I hand delivered the manuscript to Frank, I remarked to Chuck, who had accompanied me: "I feel like I just delivered a baby—my first book."

The downward spiral of the marriage was completed with the separation process begun and then finalized. It was not easy because of the children, at the time aged six and eight, but, fortunately, after a lot of soul-searching and some outside help, we worked out a shared custody arrangement, which was not common in those days. We made a commitment that the focus of our arrangements would be the well-being of the children.

We did our best to be supportive and cooperative with each other. Despite any feelings we each may have had about the failure of our marriage, we did our best to make this new state work for all of us. We arranged to live close to each other so that the children's back-and-forth movements could take place relatively easily. They stayed in their home school. I hired students to live in with me in my newly purchased neighborhood townhouse so that they could help with driving and babysitting because of my complex work schedule. I learned to be an *adequate* cook, and followed Diti's advice to buy a microwave oven, a newly available product at the time that, despite its huge size and price, was a lifesaver. I will admit that I did almost choke Amir one evening by serving my first attempt at a roast cooked in the microwave, not realizing there was a preferable *slow-cook* mode. He started choking at the dinner table while Neta and our live-in help Fernando continued a conversation unaware of what was going on. I rushed around to Amir and performed a successful Heimlich maneuver, expelling a tough piece of roast beef across the kitchen table, at which point Neta and Fernando looked up from their conversation wondering if something was wrong.

My book, *Old Enough to Feel Better: A Medical Guide for Seniors*, was released just as the specialty of geriatric medicine was confirmed in Canada. I reveled in passing the first set of examinations for the certificate and receiving the first one of its kind while having my book released to the public at the same time.

With my separation from Yael completed, I was now an "available male." The single state presented many problems, but finding female companionship was not one of them. One of my dear friends said to me, "Michael, you are single, solvent, and straight—that is golden!" Lots of friends were "fixing me up," but I had no interest in anything permanent—I was enjoying myself too much and realizing, for the first time in my life, what sexual freedom meant. As Chuck had predicted, "getting laid" was no big deal. In fact, I was surprised by how forward women could be and how many had no interest in a permanent relationship at the time we were together. For me, this meant there could be enjoyment without feeling pressured to figure out if this was the *right one*. Traveling to conferences was especially enjoyable as there was almost always a woman who expressed an interest and sometimes boldly took the first step. I recall one meeting with a Canadian federal department in Ottawa, where, based on a second book I had written on the subject, I had been asked to provide an in-service on retirement. Sitting next to me at the dinner after the meeting was the attractive assistant to a senior bureaucrat. Enjoying a coffee after the meal, I felt her hand slip over my thigh and give it a light squeeze. I looked at her trying not to reveal my joyful and bemused surprise and grabbed her hand with my own, giving it a squeeze but removing it gently to avoid squealing or laughing publicly in delight. Despite her clearly expressed interest, it was an offer that I was too tired to accept, and, after a few phone calls from her when I returned home, it became clear that she was looking for something in a relationship I could not deliver.

Neta and Amir seemed to be coping well, and I was careful about introducing them to any of the women in my life, but could not always prevent that from happening. They knew, and seemed to understand, that, as a single person, I would be dating, as was Yael. Eventually, I began to tire of the short one- or few-night stands—even though the sex was often very exciting—and began to think about my future. Gradually, I started limiting the women I would go out with to avoid getting sidetracked from a long-term, viable relationship for which I now seemed ready. The first decision I made in this regard was not to go out with anyone who smoked—something I had informally decided previously for the purposes of personal comfort, but which now became an absolute. Then there was the Jewish factor: I figured that, even though I had gone out with and enjoyed liaisons with some wonderful non-Jewish women, over the long term, I knew that sharing the same religious practice and heritage mattered to me. The last factor was to limit my explorations to women who did not already have children but who were young enough to have a family.

That did limit my options quite a bit as I was already in my late thirties and had two children, and many of the people who were fixing me up had their divorced friends in mind.

I discovered that there were lots of Jewish women in their late twenties and early thirties who were interested in me—and my situation. On one of my trips, I had met Lisa, a resident in geriatrics from Winnipeg who, on a visit to Toronto, arranged to meet with me for coffee. Because she was visiting her sister, she asked if I would mind meeting the two of them as they had activities already booked together that Sunday. This is how I met Gilda, my wife—at the Varsity Diner on Bloor Street. Gilda was striking with her long blond hair, and our conversation focused primarily on music with the occasional refocus for Lisa's sake to the geriatric conference that had brought her to the city and which began the next day. As we got up to leave, I asked Gilda, "Maybe we could go to a concert sometime?"

"Sure, that would be very nice," she said, as she gave me her phone number.

Within a few months, I had stopped dating the other women whom I had been seeing and would sleep over at Gilda's place from time to time when I had to be downtown early in the morning and did not have Neta and Amir to look after. The children clearly liked her and her cooking, especially her version of sweet-and-sour meatballs, which she would prepare from time to time, delivering the food to the house for a meal. It was getting close to the summer. The kids were going to summer camp, and I was to be the camp doctor for two weeks. Gilda was going to a special camp not far from the kids' camp, where she was to work as a speech therapist. Before that, we went to Stratford for the weekend, and, by the end of the outing, I had been told in no uncertain terms: "This is going to be a serious relationship, or we are breaking up. I don't have the time to wait around for you to figure out what you want to do about us." I told the kids that we had broken up, and they were heartbroken. I was confused. I wasn't sure I was ready to take on a permanent relationship again. Gilda was very special, smart, insightful, beautiful, and wonderful with the children. She told me not to call unless it was to be serious.

One evening some time later, I was driving down Toronto's Bathurst Street. It was raining. I saw an old, beat-up, silver Datsun, which I recognized as Gilda's. I knew she was rehearsing with her cousin for a wedding where she was going to play the flute, the lesser of her two musical instruments, with piano being the dominant one. I stopped my car and wrote a note and left it under her wiper blade, "I miss you. May I see you?" She called to say of course I could see her, but only under one condition.

We agreed that same week that we would get married after the summer, and phoned her parents in Winnipeg and mine in New York. The summer passed. My camp experience of two weeks allowed us to get together occasionally as her camp was not that far away. When camp finished, we moved into my townhouse together and started planning the wedding. It was a challenge for her living so far north, as she had lived downtown and her work was mostly centered there. We decided that, for the sake of the children, with whom I still had shared custody, it mattered a great deal that we remain in the neighborhood so they wouldn't have to change schools.

Our wedding in Winnipeg at her parents' golf club was quite an event, with many from my family attending. We returned to Toronto, getting into the routine of married life, but decided we would like to have a house that was ours. Within a few months, we moved a couple of kilometers from where we had been living, ironically a few blocks from the last house I had shared with Yael. The kids could still attend their old school. Yael had remarried before I did, and was settled into her new life, so, for the most part, despite some glitches, we managed to be civil with each other.

Toward the spring, Gilda questioned, "How would you feel about my applying to law school? I find my job as a speech therapist with the school board boring."

"Sure, go ahead and apply." As an "emancipated" male, I felt that supporting her in this way was the "right thing to do." More importantly, it was something Gilda really wanted to do, and, without almost any preparation, she was accepted to Osgood Law School in Toronto. When she was accepted, I was not surprised, but was suddenly struck by the implications of this new undertaking. We had just bought a house, and the estimations of our ability to carry the mortgage had been based on two contributing incomes, for mine was not all that high at the time. Now there would be only my income, with additional tuition costs, to carry. Over the next three years, we were faced with a number of challenges that went with Gilda's law studies, which she enjoyed very much. We managed financially, as I was able to take on extra work to supplement our income. She wanted very much to get pregnant, but I was still reluctant to start a family. However, we decided to take our chances, and despite innumerable pregnancies that resulted in early miscarriages, it eventually happened.

One afternoon, Gilda's gynecologist advised her that, in order to become pregnant and maintain the pregnancy to term, she might consider changing her longtime practice as a lacto-ovo vegetarian. He felt that perhaps her protein intake was not adequate to sustain her pregnancies. That evening, I was surprised to see Gilda serving both steak and chicken, which was somewhat unusual even though she was in the habit of preparing meat for me, a practicing carnivore. As I was about to comment on the novelty of having both dishes presented in one meal, she picked up a T-bone steak and started gnawing on it with great relish. "If this is what I have to do to get pregnant and keep the baby, I will give it a try!" I attribute Talia to that steak. Likewise, with the pregnancy that resulted in the birth of Eytan, Gilda initiated the meat-

and-chicken regimen as soon as the pregnancy test came back positive. For us, at least, it seemed to be an inspired formula for successful pregnancies.

Talia was born on January 30, 1987, as Gilda was entering her last semester of law school. Through the combined efforts of a live-in "mother's helper" and me, we managed to support Gilda so that, even with a newborn baby, she was able to complete her studies and obtain her law degree.

"I've decided to stay home and not article (do a required law "internship" before being able to practice law) yet," she told me. I was surprised—and yet, not surprised, given how much she wanted to be a mother. It meant Gilda was home much of the day, but soon she undertook some volunteer work in a community legal clinic. Two years later, Eytan was born, and, with two children, Gilda staying home made even more sense. I continued with my career path at Baycrest and Mt. Sinai and with writing and public speaking. Talia started with the preschool and then school process, followed soon after by her brother Eytan. Seven years after completing law school, Gilda undertook part-time articling—a new option in the province—and two years later sat the bar exams becoming a licensed lawyer, ready for work, which was soon arranged in the community legal clinic in which she had previously volunteered.

Over the course of our marriage, we have experienced the usual, but often difficult, family transitions that are part of the life process: the very sad death of my mother, Neta's marriage, followed by the birth of her two daughters, the move of my father to be closer to Diti in Chicago, the decision by Amir to remain in Florida, and eventually, in the spring of 2007, my retirement from the position of vice president of medical services and head of geriatrics at Baycrest, after which I moved to a lesser role but remained at the Center.

I undertook more writing and public speaking and focused on an ethics guide for children of aging parents, a sequel to my book released in 2001, *Parenting Your Parents*, which was coauthored by Bart Mindszenthy (with whom I have developed a wonderful working relationship). Both the book and the subsequent speaking engagements that followed its release opened new avenues of professional adventure for me, which proved, and continue to be, satisfying and enjoyable.

This book of reflections you are reading now records my personal odyssey through the world of medicine. It captures selected experiences of my past life that might be shared, and hopefully enjoyed, by family, friends, colleagues, and a general readership interested in events in the development of the world of aging. Whether my life story has any monumental significance was not the point: I thought that, even if I touched one person in sharing the many experiences of my life, then the book would have been worth the effort. The writing of this story has been personally rewarding as it has allowed me not just to reexperience the past, but to come to an understanding of how it has contributed to making me the man I am today. In so doing, I recognize that life has been very good to me. I feel very fortunate, and have found enormous fulfillment and joy in sharing that life with the many people with whom I have had the privilege, both personal and professional, to walk this journey.

L'Chaim!